Airway Reconstruction
Surgical Dissection Manual

Airway Reconstruction Surgical Dissection Manual

Evan J. Propst, MD, MSc, FRCSC
Yamilet Tirado, MD
Faisal I. Abdulkader, BM, MSc, FRCS
Marvin Estrada, VT
Paolo Campisi, MSc, MD, FRCSC, FAAP
Vito Forte, MD, FRCSC

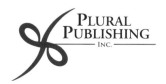

PLURAL
PUBLISHING
INC.

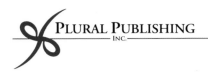

5521 Ruffin Road
San Diego, CA 92123

e-mail: info@pluralpublishing.com
Website: http://www.pluralpublishing.com

NOTICE TO THE READER
Care has been taken to confirm the accuracy of the indications, procedures, drug dosages, and diagnosis and remediation protocols presented in this book and to ensure that they conform to the practices of the general medical and health services communities. However, the authors, editors, and publisher are not responsible for errors or omissions or for any consequences from application of the information in this book and make no warranty, expressed or implied, with respect to the currency, completeness, or accuracy of the contents of the publication. The diagnostic and remediation protocols and the medications described do not necessarily have specific approval by the Food and Drug Administration for use in the disorders and/or diseases and dosages for which they are recommended. Application of this information in a particular situation remains the professional responsibility of the practitioner. Because standards of practice and usage change, it is the responsibility of the practitioner to keep abreast of revised recommendations, dosages, and procedures.

Library of Congress Cataloging-in-Publication Data

Propst, Evan J., author.
  Airway reconstruction surgical dissection manual / Evan J. Propst [and 5 others].
    p. ; cm.
  Includes bibliographical references and index.
  ISBN-13: 978-1-59756-572-1 (alk. paper)
  ISBN-10: 1-59756-572-5 (alk. paper)
  I. Title.
  [DNLM: 1. Trachea—surgery. 2. Dissection—methods. 3. Reconstructive Surgical Procedures—methods. 4. Swine. 5. Trachea—anatomy & histology. WF 490]
  RD536
  617.5'4—dc23
                                                              2013039356

Contents

Note: Animals used in these dissections are Yorkshire pigs. All photos are taken with the surgeon standing on the pig's right side unless otherwise specified.

Foreword

It is with great pleasure that I write this foreword. This takes me personally back to 1970 when my mentor Dr. Fearon and I were researching surgical techniques for reconstruction of the pediatric airway using African green monkeys as our operative model. The term "translational" research was not current at that time but this indeed was a great example of this. I also did not realize that this would lead to my chosen career path in the future. The need for such work arose because of the emergence of a new disease entity in infants following the introduction of long-term intubation as a means of respiratory support in premature infants, leading to the development of subglottic stenosis and tracheotomy in an unfortunate few. The outcome of this work was that the Cotton anterior graft reconstruction became the standard workhorse of airway surgery in children.

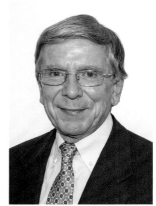

Robin T. Cotton

The senior author, Evan Propst, was a fellow in our Division at Cincinnati Children's Hospital (CCHMC) from 2008 to 2010 and became thoroughly exposed to all the techniques of pediatric airway surgery that have developed over the past 45 years. Concurrently, Evan was exposed to several members of our Division who were developing a curriculum for simulation in pediatric otolaryngologic procedures in general, including airway surgery. The synergism of this exposure to live surgical procedures and simulation has led to his development of this most important text.

This cutting-edge manual is a supreme example of being the right publication at the right time. It will be of great benefit not only to all trainees in pediatric otolaryngology but also worldwide to younger and midlevel specialists who may not have had in-depth exposure to airway surgery in their training yet who are in a position to treat these patients in their local environments. This manual fills a niche that is presently empty. As I read the chapter on harvest of costal cartilage, I recalled that while doing my first costal cartilage harvest in the operating room at CCHMC in 1974, I was confronted by one of my pediatric surgical colleagues "offering his help" as needed. I have to feel this book would have increased my confidence level at that moment!

In summary, this beautifully written and illustrated book will be of great importance to all pediatric otolaryngologists worldwide who treat children with airway problems. Following the guidelines will enable the practitioner to test his or her surgical skills prior to the operating room. This will be a classic for many years to come.

Robin T. Cotton, MD, FACS, FRCSC
Director
Aerodigestive and Sleep Center
Cincinnati Children's Hospital Medical Center
Professor
Department of Otolaryngology-Head and Neck Surgery
Department of Pediatrics
University of Cincinnati College of Medicine
Cincinnati, United States of America

Foreword

It is a pleasure to have been invited to write the foreword to this very timely manual that covers the historical developments and current approaches to, and techniques for repairing simple to complex defects of laryngotracheal stenosis. The collective experience of the authors is beyond question, because they are the products of the learning curve that I have had a unique opportunity to be part of during the past 30 years.

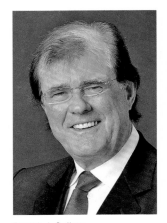

Patrick J. Gullane

This manual demonstrates a variety of techniques in a most detailed descriptive manner that will help our trainees to better understand the menu of approaches in each selective type of problem. The material is presented in a most clear and concise manner that includes critical and contrasting points of view. This text chronicles the breadth and depth of understanding necessary to optimize the best result when selecting the most appropriate technique, as shown by the authors. This publication is a major contribution to this poorly understood area, and in my opinion should be compulsory reading for our residents and fellows in training.

This work is a timely account of the current knowledge of airway repair. I congratulate the editors for their vision and creativity in preparing this comprehensive reference text.

Patrick J. Gullane, CM, MB, FRCSC, FACS, FRACS(Hon), FRCS(Hon), FRCSI(Hon)
Wharton Chair in Head and Neck Surgery
Professor
Department of Otolaryngology-Head and Neck Surgery
Department of Surgery
University of Toronto
Toronto, Canada

Foreword

The authors of this surgical dissection manual must be congratulated for providing a useful adjunct to the field of pediatric airway reconstruction. The idea of describing the surgical steps of each procedure in detail in a porcine model will be invaluable for all surgeons wishing to gain a basic understanding of, and surgical skills in, this field.

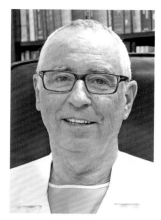

Philippe Monnier

Each chapter is richly illustrated and concisely written in a step-by-step manner. The high-quality operative views with only essential descriptions added render the comprehension of each procedure both simple and clear. All basic airway reconstructions such as anterior cricoid split, harvest of thyroid and costal cartilages, tracheotomy, different LTRs, CTR, and slide tracheoplasty are clearly described.

This book will undoubtedly stand as a first approach to pediatric airway reconstruction surgery and belongs on the bookshelf of all junior surgeons wishing to develop their surgical skills prior to operating on human beings.

Philippe Monnier, MD
Professor Emeritus
Department of Otolaryngology-Head and Neck Surgery
School of Biology and Medicine
University of Lausanne
Lausanne, Switzerland

Preface

Exposure to open airway surgery is often limited during Otolaryngology residency and is variable and often inadequate in many Pediatric Otolaryngology fellowship programs. This is largely due to a decrease in the number of patients with subglottic stenosis (due to a better awareness of the injurious effects of endotracheal tube cuffs and the drastic reduction of infectious diseases such as diphtheria) and is further compounded by new Resident work hour restrictions. As a result, Residency and Fellowship programs must develop surgical simulation models to ensure that trainees become proficient in open airway surgery.

As you work through this surgical manual, the contributions of many great surgeons will become evident. It is interesting to follow the evolution of thought over time that led to the surgeries that are presently considered to be the standard of care. We highlight here some of the major contributions in the field of open airway surgery.

The first description of the anterior cricoid split appears in the early 1900s by Killian (Germany) and the first description of the posterior cricoid split is credited to Galebsky (Lenningrad) in 1927.[1,2] In 1938, Looper (Baltimore) rotated the hyoid bone to augment a stenotic adult laryngeal fracture sustained in a railroad accident.[3] In 1968, Lapidot (New York) used this principle in piglets to show that a flap of thyroid cartilage rotated on perichondrium to replace a segment of resected cricoid cartilage could survive, suggesting that laryngeal growth could continue after reconstruction without restenosis.[4]

Great advances in open airway reconstruction were made in the 1970s, many of which occurred in Toronto, Canada. In 1971, Fearon and Ellis described a child with severe subglottic stenosis who, after failed dilatations and anterior cricoid split with auricular cartilage graft augmentation, eventually underwent tracheotomy, placement of an anterior costal cartilage graft with buccal mucosa and a stent and was eventually decannulated.[5] Fearon and Cotton further investigated tracheal augmentation using thyroid cartilage (harvested from the inferior border) in African green monkeys and proved that the cricoid could be divided without inhibition of laryngeal growth.[6] In 1976, Fearon and Cinnamond reported on 35 patients operated on using this technique between 1970 and 1976, noting that free thyroid grafts were more feasible than pedicled grafts and that costal cartilage was most suitable for repairing long segment stenoses.[7] They also proposed that shaping anterior costal cartilage grafts with flanges might prevent them from being displaced inward into the trachea.[7] Cotton would later be the first to describe in detail the process of harvesting, carving and insetting an anterior costal cartilage graft along with his success using this technique in 11 children after moving to Cincinnati.[8] In 1973, Crysdale visited Grahne in Helsinki, Finland, to observe an anterior-posterior cricoid split with stent placement and was the first to perform this procedure in a child in North America.[9,10] A search for less morbid sources of cartilage for anterior cricoid augmentation in neonates allowed Park and Forte (1999) to demonstrate that bilateral cartilaginous grafts could be harvested from the superior aspect of the thyroid cartilage in kittens without airway compromise. Success using this technique was later demonstrated in 2001 by Forte, Chang, and Papsin in a series of 17 children.[11,12] For more severe subglottic stenoses, Gerwat and Bryce (1974) described the first cricotracheal resection with preservation of the recurrent laryngeal nerves. Conley (1956) included this surgery in his list of ways to reconstruct the subglottic air passage but gave no details of his experience; whereas, Ogura and Powers (1964) described this

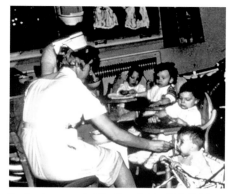

Tracheotomy ward at the Hospital for Sick Children in early 1970s. Photo taken by Blair Fearon, courtesy Robin Cotton.

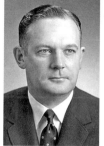

Dr. Blair Fearon

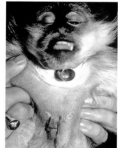

African green monkey with tracheotomy following open airway surgery. Photo courtesy Robin Cotton.

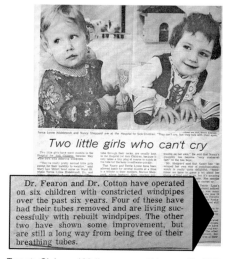

Toronto Globe and Mail newspaper, February 12, 1977

Preface

procedure in patients with previous bilateral vocal fold paralysis.[13–15] Pearson and Gullane would later report their success using this procedure over the ensuing 22 years in 80 consecutive adults with benign subglottic stenosis.[16] Impressed by the results of Gerwat and Bryce, Monnier, Savary, and Chapuis (Lausanne, Switzerland) performed the first cricoid resection with primary anastomosis in a child in 1978.[17]

Even though many of these innovations are considered to be the framework for present-day open airway reconstruction, it is important to recognize that there are as many variations in technique as there are surgeons performing these procedures. While this manual does not delve into the many variations of each technique, it does provide a very detailed way of performing each type of open airway surgery based on techniques learned while training in both Toronto and Cincinnati. It is incumbent upon the trainee to be creative and improve upon these surgeries in the future.

We hope you enjoy working through this manual as much as we enjoyed creating it.

Sincerely,
Evan J. Propst, MD

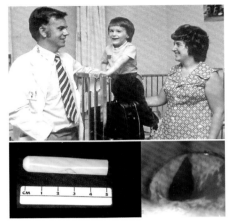

William Crysdale with first patient to undergo anterior-posterior cricoid split prior to discharge, July 1974. Actual Aboulker stent used in this patient (*bottom left*). Patient larynx, September 1975 (*bottom right*). Photos courtesy William Crysdale.

References

1. Winslow JR. Report of cases illustrating our progress in the surgical treatment of chronic stenosis of the larynx and trachea. *Laryngoscope*. 1909;19:773–784.
2. Rethi A. An operation for cicatricial stenosis of the larynx. *J Laryngol Otol*. 1956;70(5):283–293.
3. Looper EA. Use of the hyoid bone as a graft in laryngeal stenosis. *Arch Otolaryngol*. 1938;28:106-111.
4. Lapidot A, Sodagar R, Ratanaprashtporn S, Silverman R. Experimental repair of subglottic stenosis in piglets: "Trapdoor" thyrochondroplasty flap. *Arch Laryngol*. 1968;88:529–535.
5. Fearon B, Ellis D. The management of long term airway problems in infants and children. *Ann Otol Rhinol Laryngol*. 1971;80:669–677.
6. Fearon B, Cotton R. Surgical correction of subglottic stenosis of the larynx: preliminary report of an experimental surgical technique. *Ann Otol Rhinol Laryngol*. 1972;81:508–513.
7. Fearon B, Cinnamond M. Surgical correction of subglottic stenosis of the larynx: clinical results of the Fearon-Cotton operation. *J Otolaryngol*. 1976;5:475–478.
8. Cotton R. Management of subglottic stenosis in infancy and childhood: review of a consecutive series of cases managed by surgical reconstruction. *Ann Otol Rhinol Laryngol*. 1978;87:649–657.
9. Crysdale WS. Extended laryngofissure in the management of subglottic stenosis in the young child: a preliminary report. *J Otolaryngol*. 1976;5:479–486.
10. Crysdale WS, Platt LJ. Division of posterior cricoid plate in young children with subglottic stenosis. *Laryngoscope*. 1976;86:1451–1458.
11. Park AH, Forte V. Effect of harvesting autogenous laryngeal cartilage for laryngotracheal reconstruction on laryngeal growth and support. *Laryngoscope*. 1999;109:307–311.
12. Forte C, Chang MB, Papsin BC. Thyroid ala cartilage reconstruction in neonatal subglottic stenosis as a replacement for the anterior cricoid split. *Int J Pediatr Otorhinolaryngol*. 2001;59:181–186.
13. Gerwat J, Bryce DP. The management of subglottic laryngeal stenosis by resection and direct anastomosis. *Laryngoscope*. 1974;84:940–957.
14. Conley JJ. Reconstruction of the subglottic air passage. *Ann Otol Rhinol Laryngol*. 1953;62:477–495.
15. Ogura JH, Powers WE. Functional restitution of traumatic stenosis of the larynx and pharynx. *Trans Am Laryngol Rhinol Otol Soc*. 1964;44:755–784.
16. Pearson FG, Gullane P. Subglottic resection with primary tracheal anastomosis: including synchronous laryngotracheal reconstructions. *Semin Thorac Cardiovasc Surg*. 1996;8:381–391.
17. Monnier P, Savary M, Chapuis G. Partial cricoid resection with primary tracheal anastomosis for subglottic stenosis in infants and children. *Laryngoscope*. 1993;103:1273–1283.

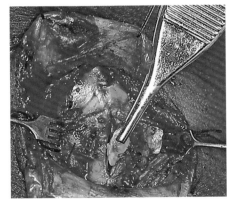

First thyroid ala graft. Photo courtesy Vito Forte.

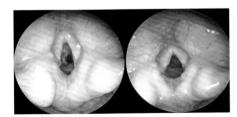

First partial cricotracheal resection in a child. Pre-operatively (*left*) and postoperatively (*right*). Photo courtesy Philippe Monnier.

Acknowledgments

We are most grateful to the staff in the Lab Animal Services for caring for the pigs used in these dissections. I am indebted to my mentors in airway surgery in Toronto (Patrick Gullane and Vito Forte) and Cincinnati (Robin Cotton, Charles Myer III, Michael Rutter, Ravindhra Elluru, Alessandro de Alarcón, Sally Shott, and J. Paul Willging), for developing and imparting the knowledge described in this book. I am indebted to Blake Papsin for being an outstanding mentor, motivator, colleague, and friend. I will always be grateful to Diana Alli and Anna Jarvis for selflessly opening doors for me. Most importantly, this work could not be completed without the unconditional support of my family: Tali, Elle, Emma, Isobel, Steve, Lara, Trevor, Anna, and Michael—thank you.

—*Evan J. Propst*

1

Introduction

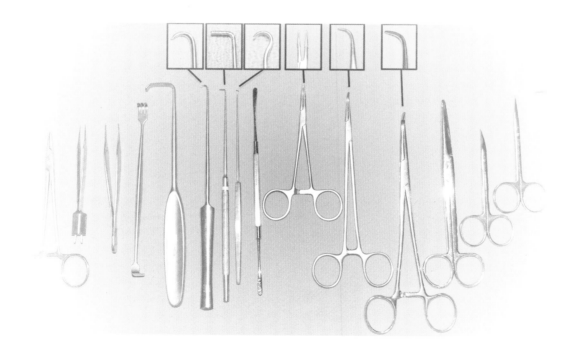

Essential
Sand bag (1)
Disposable razor (1)
Scalpel handle (1)
Needle driver (1)
Microbipolar cautery (1)
Toothed forcep (2)
Seine retractor (2)
Right-angle retractor (2)
Cricoid hook (1)
Nerve hook, blunt (2)
Skin hook (1)
Freer elevator (1)
Mosquito snap (8-10, 2 with rubber shods)
Mixter/Lauer (1)
Scissors, Mayo (1)
Scissors, Iris, straight and curved (1)
Metal cup (1)
Suction (1)

Helpful
Electric razor (1)
McGowan needle (1)
Caliper (1)
Round knife (1)
Ribbon retractor (2)
Self-retaining retractor (1)
Jake dissector (1)
Towel clip (4)

Optional
Otologic drill
Flexible bronchoscope
Rigid bronchoscope

Procurement, Transport, and Housing of Animals

We find that piglets weighing 10 to 15 kg are the ideal size for airway surgical dissection. Pigs arrive at the facility one day prior to surgery and are fasted overnight. They are housed two pigs per cage.

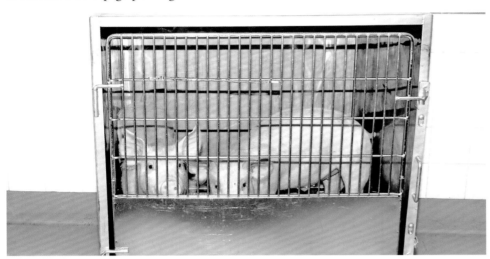

Operating Room Setup

At minimum, you will need an operating table, anesthetic machine, overhead lighting, a table to hold your instruments, and a waste bin.

KEY POINTS
Operating table
Anesthetic machine
Overhead lighting
Table for instruments
Waste bin

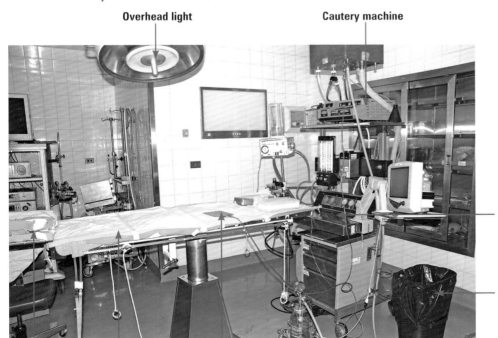

Overhead light   Cautery machine

Anesthestic machine

Waste bin

Table for instruments   Operating table   Grounding pad for monopolar cautery

Surgical Instruments

Essential

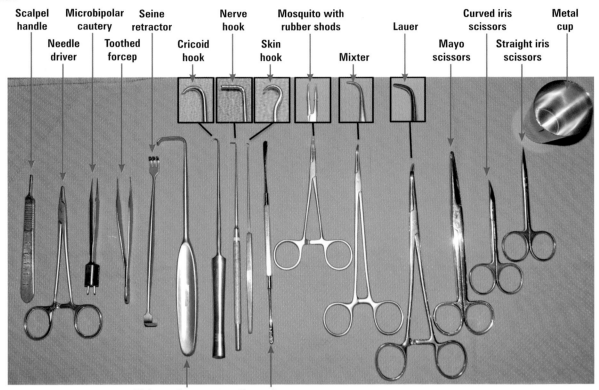

Scalpel handle · Needle driver · Microbipolar cautery · Toothed forcep · Seine retractor · Cricoid hook · Nerve hook · Skin hook · Mosquito with rubber shods · Mixter · Lauer · Mayo scissors · Curved iris scissors · Straight iris scissors · Metal cup

Right-angle retractor · Freer elevator

Helpful

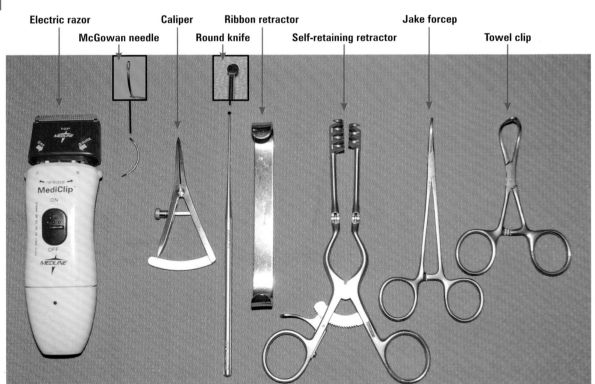

Electric razor · McGowan needle · Caliper · Round knife · Ribbon retractor · Self-retaining retractor · Jake forcep · Towel clip

2

Induction of Anesthesia and Intubation

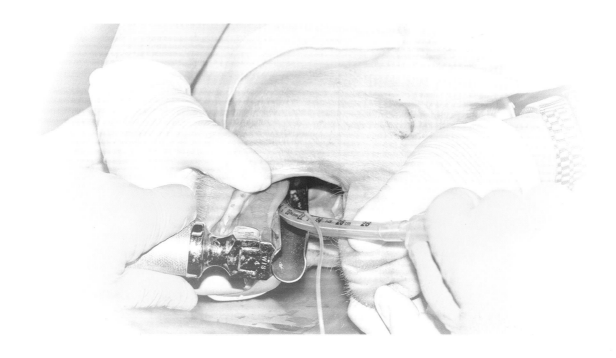

Disposable Items You Will Need

MEDICATIONS

- Akmezine
- Normal saline bag (3)

SHARPS

- 16- or 18-Gauge angiocatheter (1)
- 25-Gauge Butterfly needle (1)

OTHER

- 10 mL syringe (1)
- Intravenous tubing (1)
- 6.0 or 6.5 Cuffed endotracheal tube (1)
- Gloves (2 pairs)
- Strip of material (30 cm)
- Absorbent pad (1)
- Rope (180 cm)

OPTIONAL

- None

Induction of Anesthesia and Intubation

At our facility, a veterinarian is present at all times to assist with preoperative care, anesthesia, euthanasia, and medical emergencies.

Step 1 Each pig is premedicated with Akmezine 0.16 to 0.20 mL/kg. (Each mL of Akmezine contains 58.82 mg ketamine, 1.18 mg acepromazine, and 0.09 mg atropine.) Place this mixture in a syringe with intravenous tubing and a butterfly needle on the end. Skillfully place the needle intramuscularly into the pig's neck and inject the medication. Wait approximately 15 to 20 minutes for the medication to take effect.

KEY POINTS

Premedicate with Akmezine

Butterfly needle into neck

Wait 15 to 20 minutes

Induce with isoflurane and oxygen

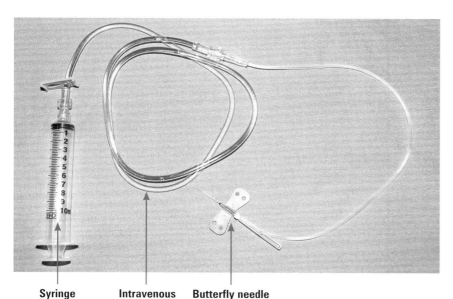
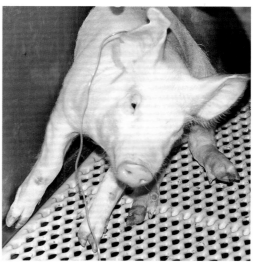

Syringe **Intravenous tubing** **Butterfly needle**

Step 2 Place the pig on the operating table and put the mask over its snout. Anesthesia is induced with 3 to 4% isoflurane mixed with 2 L oxygen.

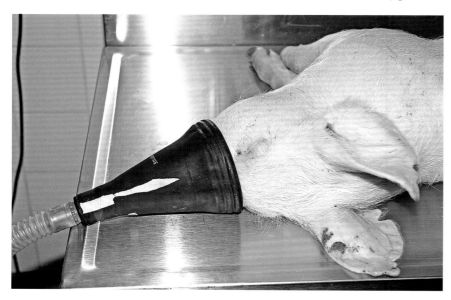

Induction of Anesthesia and Intubation

2

Step 3 The laryngoscope used to intubate a piglet is much longer than that used for humans. Generally, piglets that are 10 to 15 kg require either a 6.0 or 6.5 cuffed endotracheal tube.

KEY POINTS

6.0 or 6.5 cuffed endotracheal tube

Two-person technique

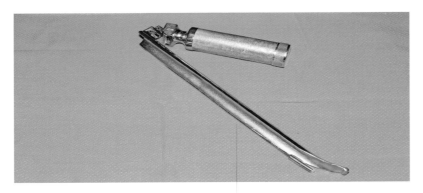

Step 4 We use a two-person technique to intubate pigs. The first person (white gloves) grasps the snout with one hand and opens the jaw with the other. The second person (blue gloves) inserts the laryngoscope to push the tongue inferiorly until the epiglottis and glottis are seen. The epiglottis must be dropped below the soft palate to expose the larynx in the pig. The second person intubates the pig. Secure the tube in place with a strip of material by tying a knot around the tube and then another around the snout.

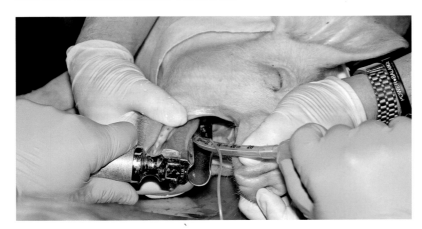

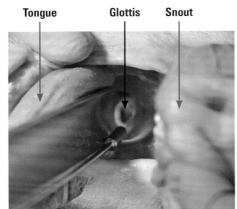
Tongue   Glottis   Snout

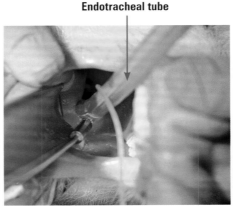
Endotracheal tube

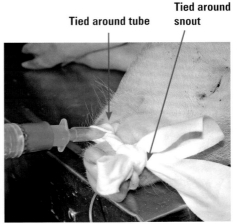
Tied around tube   Tied around snout

Step 5 Tape an absorbent pad around the lower end of the pig to collect urine and feces.

KEY POINTS

Absorbent pad on lower end of pig

Sand bag under shoulders

Secure pig to table with rope

Cautery grounding pad   Secure arms to table with rope   Sand bag under shoulders   Absorbent pad

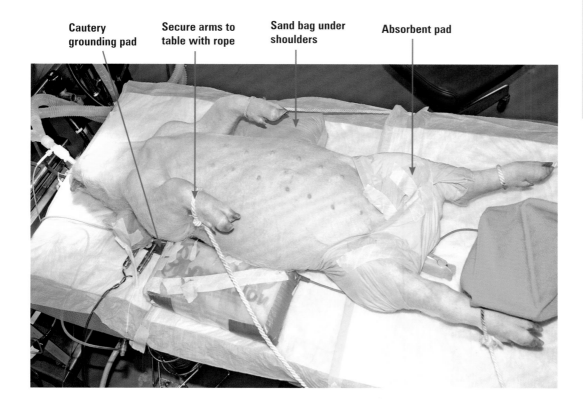

Step 6 Place a sand bag under the shoulders to lift the trachea anteriorly for easier exposure.

Step 7 Secure the pig's arms to the table with rope.

Step 8   Place an intravenous catheter (16- or 18-gauge) in an ear vein and tape it in place. Deliver normal saline through this intravenous at a rate of 70 mL/h.

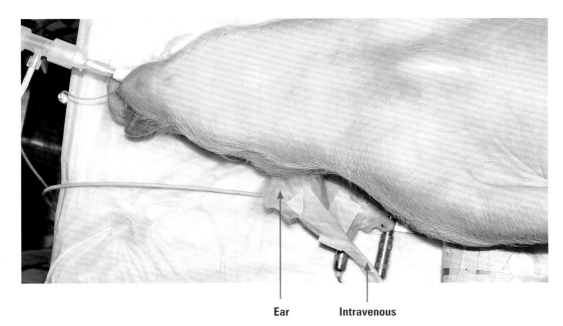

Ear   Intravenous

Step 9   Shave the tail and place an oxygen saturation monitor on it.

Tail   Absorbent pad

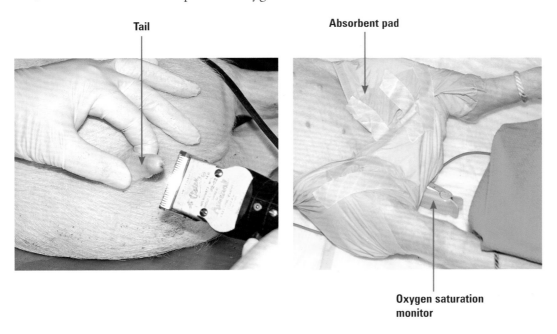

Oxygen saturation monitor

Step 10   Place an electrocautery grounding pad on the pig's back.

3

Exposure and Anatomy of the Pig Airway

Comparison with the Human Airway

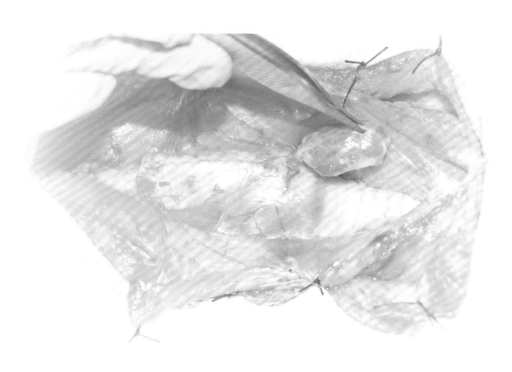

Disposable Items You Will Need

MEDICATIONS

- Akmezine
- Normal saline bag (3)

SHARPS

- 16- or 18-Gauge angiocatheter (1)
- 25-Gauge Butterfly needle (1)
- 2-0 Silk suture (6)
- #15 Blade (1)

OTHER

- 10 mL syringe (1)
- Intravenous tubing (1)
- 6.0 or 6.5 Cuffed endotracheal tube (1)
- Gloves (2 pairs)
- Strip of material (30 cm)
- Absorbent pad (1)
- Rope (180 cm)
- Marking pen (1)
- Ruler (1)
- Green towel (4)

OPTIONAL

- None

Exposure and Anatomy of the Pig Airway: Comparison with the Human Airway

3

There are many similarities in the anatomy of the head and neck in pigs and humans making the pig an excellent surgical training model. However, attention should be paid to minor differences to allow for successful training on this porcine model and appropriate translation of surgical skills to humans. For ease of understanding, comparisons between pigs and humans will be *italicized* throughout the text.

We do not routinely sterily prepare the surgical site prior to surgery if the pig is to be euthanized at the end of the procedure. If the pig is to be survived for experimental reasons, it will be prepped with Betadine from the snout to the chest. *In humans, we prepare the surgical site(s) with Betadine and perform the surgery under sterile conditions.*

Step 1   Place green towels around the surgical site and hold them in place with towel clamps.

Step 2   Mark the most prominent part of the thyroid cartilage and the sternal notch. Draw a vertical line connecting the two and extend this line 4 cm superior to the thyroid cartilage *(to the level of the hyoid bone, which is difficult to palpate in pigs). In humans, a horizontal incision is made in a neck crease and subplatysmal flaps are raised superiorly to the level of the hyoid bone and inferiorly to the clavicles. The pig's thick tissues make it difficult to raise subplatysmal flaps superiorly and inferiorly.*

Thyroid cartilage   Sternal notch

4 cm

Exposure and Anatomy of the Pig Airway: Comparison with the Human Airway

3

Step 3 Use a #15 blade to make a vertical incision through the skin.

Step 4 Use microbipolar cautery to divide the platysma vertically if it is present.

Step 5 Elevate subplatysmal flaps laterally.

Step 6 Suture the flaps laterally to the skin using 2-0 silk sutures for exposure. *In humans, we prefer to tie the sutures to the drapes as this is less traumatic.* This exposes the vertical strap muscles.

KEY POINTS

Vertical skin incision

Elevate subplatysmal flaps

Suture laterally

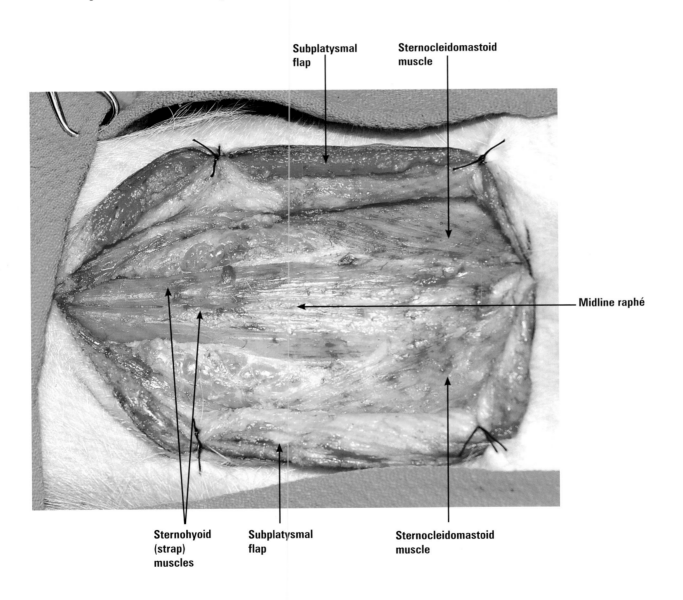

Subplatysmal flap

Sternocleidomastoid muscle

Midline raphé

Sternohyoid (strap) muscles

Subplatysmal flap

Sternocleidomastoid muscle

Step 7   Divide the sternohyoid (strap) muscles in the midline superiorly up to the hyoid bone and inferiorly down to the sternal notch. Suture them to the skin laterally for retraction. Gently place a finger posterior to the sternal notch to palpate for the innominate artery (brachiocephalic artery) to ensure it is not injured while dividing the strap muscles inferiorly. Retraction of the sternohyoid muscles exposes the sternothyroid muscles.

KEY POINTS

Divide sternohyoid muscles

Palpate for innominate artery

Expose sternothyroid muscles

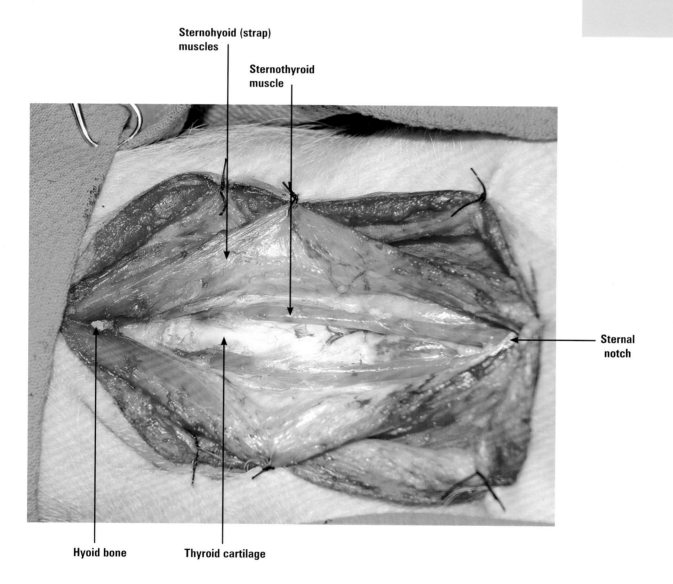

Sternohyoid (strap) muscles

Sternothyroid muscle

Sternal notch

Hyoid bone

Thyroid cartilage

Step 8 Peel the sternothyroid muscles off the laryngeal and tracheal cartilages and suture them to the skin laterally for retraction. *In the pig, there is an extra set of vertical muscles that run from the sternum to the thyroid cartilage and then to the cricoid (that we have named sternothyrocricoid muscles) that are not present in humans but nevertheless need to be retracted.*

Sternothyroid muscles

Sternothyrocricoid muscles

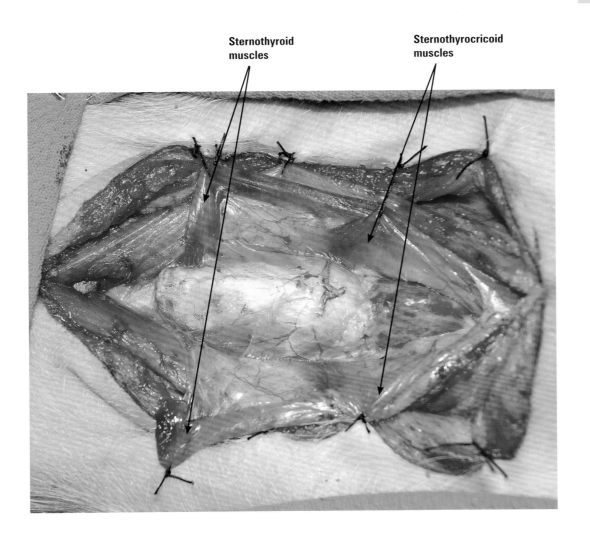

Step 9 Remove the thyroid gland to expose the cricoid and trachea. *In humans, the thyroid gland is NOT removed. The human thyroid gland lies lower in the neck and therefore does not usually interfere with visualization of the airway. If the surgeon decides that the thyroid gland absolutely has to be moved to perform the surgery, the thyroid isthmus is divided in the midline to gain access to the trachea. Note the thyroid cartilage in the pig, which does not have a notch (human thyroid cartilage has a notch) and the cricothyroid muscles (humans have a thinner membrane rather than thicker muscles). The thyroid and cricoid cartilages are more anterior than the trachea in the pig as compared with humans, in whom they are not. This makes it more difficult to perform a laryngotracheoplasty with placement of an anterior graft in this porcine model.*

KEY POINTS

Thyroid gland removed in pigs only

Absent thyroid notch

Cricothyroid muscles rather than membrane

During Removal of Thyroid Gland

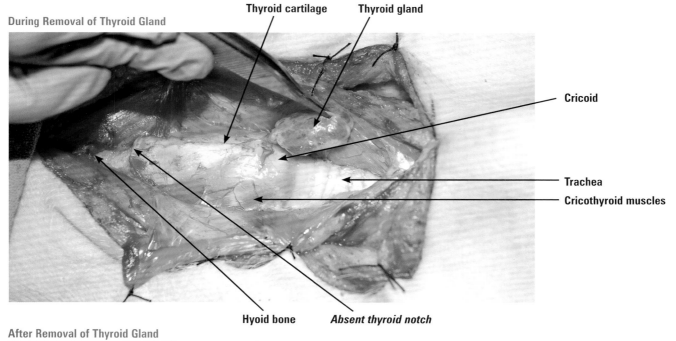

Thyroid cartilage   Thyroid gland

Cricoid

Trachea
Cricothyroid muscles

Hyoid bone   *Absent thyroid notch*

After Removal of Thyroid Gland

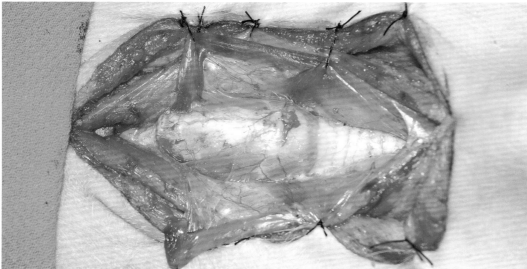

4

Anterior Cricoid Split (Single Stage)

Disposable Items You Will Need

MEDICATIONS

- Akmezine
- Normal saline bag (3)

SHARPS

- 16- or 18-Gauge angiocatheter (1)
- 25-Gauge Butterfly needle (1)
- 2-0 Silk suture (6)
- #15 Blade (1)

OTHER

- 10 mL syringe (1)
- Intravenous tubing (1)
- 6.0 or 6.5 Cuffed endotracheal tube (1)
- Gloves (2 pairs)
- Strip of material (30 cm)
- Absorbent pad (1)
- Rope (180 cm)
- Marking pen (1)
- Ruler (1)
- Green towel (4)

OPTIONAL

- None

Anterior Cricoid Split (Single Stage)

Follow the steps outlined in "Exposure and Anatomy of the Pig Airway: Comparison with the Human Airway" prior to performing this procedure.

Performing an anterior cricoid split is slightly more difficult in the pig than it is in humans because the thyroid cartilage of the pig is shaped triangularly at its inferior aspect as a condensation of the cricothyroid muscle medially and hangs over the cricoid cartilage (demarcated between scalpel handles).

KEY POINTS

Thyroid cartilage hangs over cricoid cartilage in the pig

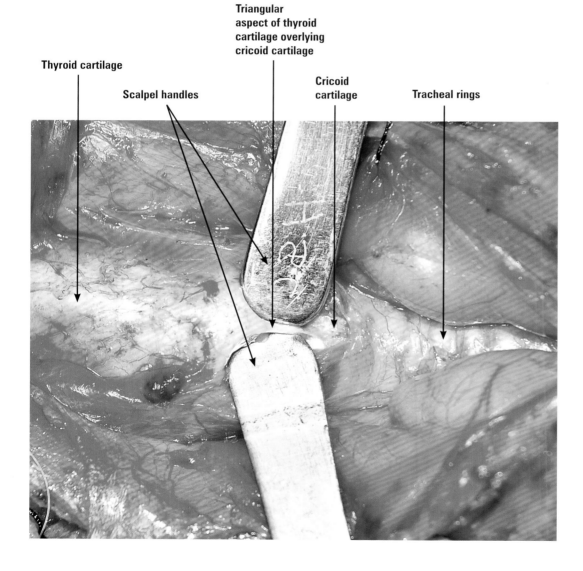

Thyroid cartilage

Scalpel handles

Triangular aspect of thyroid cartilage overlying cricoid cartilage

Cricoid cartilage

Tracheal rings

Step 1 Use a marking pen to draw a vertical line over the midline of the cricoid cartilage and the first tracheal ring. If the cricothyroid muscles obscure the midline of the cricoid cartilage, use an elevator to move them a few millimeters laterally to expose the midline of the cricoid cartilage.

KEY POINTS

Draw vertical line over midline of cricoid cartilage and first tracheal ring

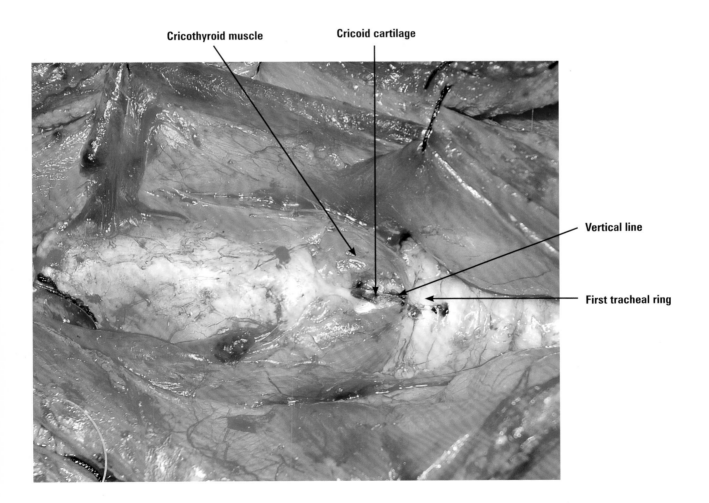

Cricothyroid muscle

Cricoid cartilage

Vertical line

First tracheal ring

Step 2 Use a #15 scalpel to divide the cricoid cartilage (Figure 1) and the first tracheal ring (Figure 2). *Because the thyroid cartilage, the cricoid cartilage, and the first tracheal ring all overlap in the pig, it helps to retract the first tracheal ring inferiorly to expose and incise the cricoid cartilage.* Similarly, retracting the thyroid cartilage superiorly with a cricoid hook (Figure 3) makes it easier to evaluate the size of the defect. Use Seine retractors to expose the tracheal lumen (Figure 4).

KEY POINTS

Divide cricoid cartilage and first tracheal ring

Retract as required to overcome limitations due to overlapping cartilages in the pig

Cut cricoid cartilage

Figure 1

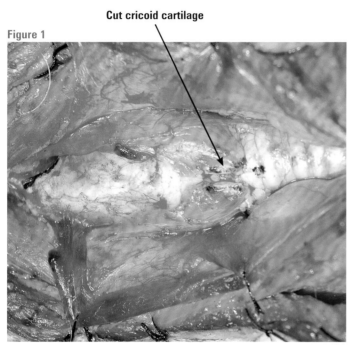

Cut first tracheal ring

Figure 2

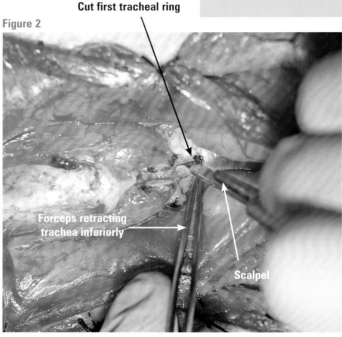

Forceps retracting trachea inferiorly

Scalpel

Figure 3

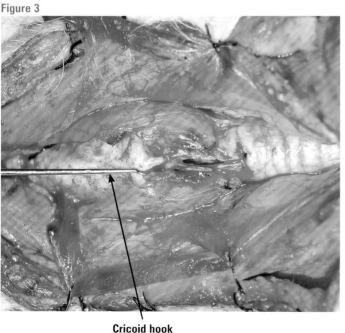

Cricoid hook

Figure 4

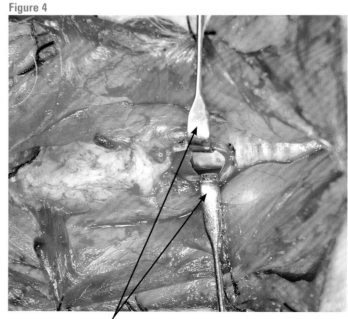

Seine retractors exposing the tracheal lumen

5

Harvest of Thyroid Ala Cartilage Graft

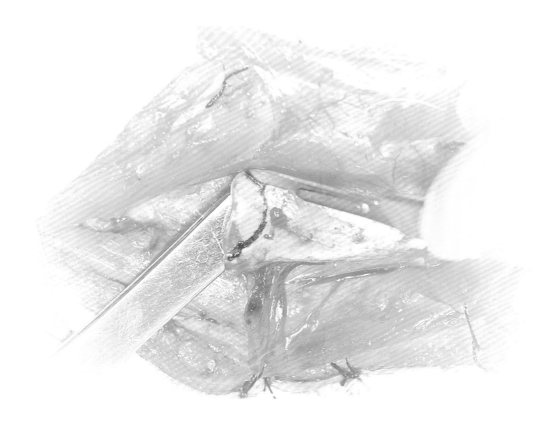

Disposable Items You Will Need

MEDICATIONS

- Akmezine
- Normal saline bag (3)

SHARPS

- 16- or 18-Gauge angiocatheter (1)
- 25-Gauge Butterfly needle (1)
- 2-0 Silk suture (6)
- #15 Blade (1)

OTHER

- 10 mL syringe (1)
- Intravenous tubing (1)
- 6.0 or 6.5 Cuffed endotracheal tube (1)
- Gloves (2 pairs)
- Strip of material (30 cm)
- Absorbent pad (1)
- Rope (180 cm)
- Marking pen (1)
- Ruler (1)
- Green towel (4)

OPTIONAL

- None

Follow the steps outlined in "Exposure and Anatomy of the Pig Airway: Comparison with the Human Airway" prior to performing this procedure.

It is usually easier for the right-handed surgeon to harvest the graft from the left thyroid ala; however, either side or both sides can be harvested. We describe here how to harvest the left thyroid ala while standing on the right side of the patient.

Step 1 Place a cricoid hook into the midline of the superior aspect of the thyroid cartilage and retract toward the right side of the pig. This maneuver holds the cartilage steady when you mark your incision. *In humans, place the cricoid hook in the thyroid notch.*

Step 2 Use a marking pen to drop a semicircle from the superior edge of the thyroid cartilage. *In humans, placing the anterior aspect of this semicircle posterior to the edge of the thyroid notch will allow male patients to develop a prominent "Adam's apple" when they reach puberty.*

KEY POINTS

Retract thyroid cartilage

Drop semicircle

Mark incision posterior to thyroid notch in humans

Superior edge of thyroid cartilage   **Semicircle**

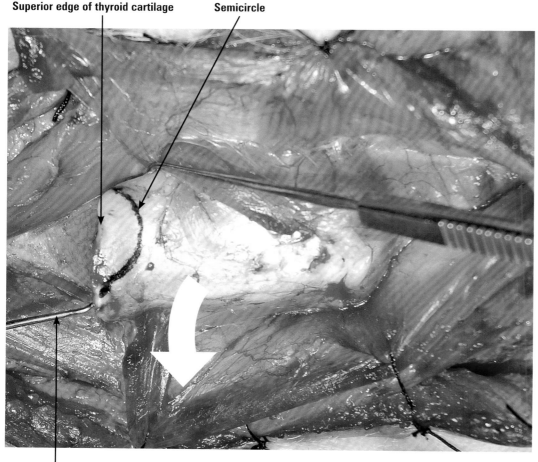

View while standing on the right side of the pig with thyroid cartilage rotated to the pig's right

Cricoid hook   **White arrow shows rolled over cartilage**

Step 3 Incise the perichondrium along the superior border of the thyroid cartilage.

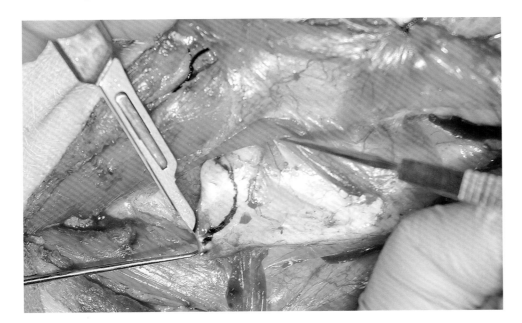

Step 4 Walk around the table and stand on the left side of the pig. Use an elevator to elevate a subperichondrial flap off the posterior aspect of the thyroid cartilage. Elevate down to the inferior border of your planned incision. Try not to perforate through the subperichondrium into the larynx. *In humans, it is easier to preserve the perichondrium on the inner surface of the cartilage and place it facing the lumen during reconstruction.*

Inferior border of planned incision

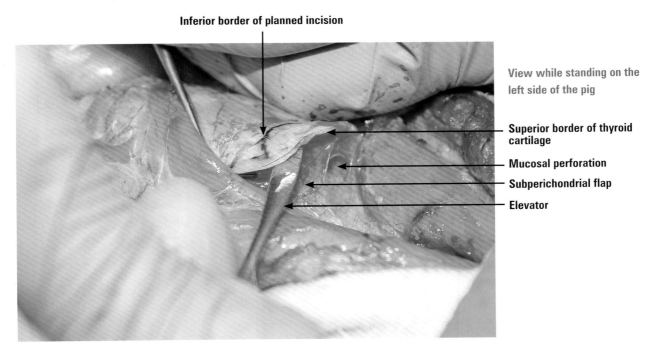

View while standing on the left side of the pig

Superior border of thyroid cartilage

Mucosal perforation

Subperichondrial flap

Elevator

Step 5 Walk back around the table and stand on the pig's right side. Place the handle of a scalpel medial to the thyroid cartilage to protect the posterior perichondrium from injury. Cut along the marked semicircle while you are pressing onto the scalpel handle with your scalpel blade.

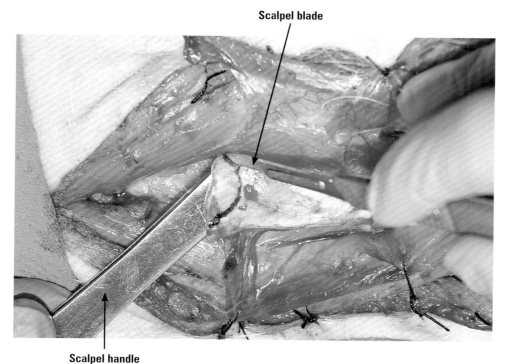

Scalpel blade

Scalpel handle

View while standing on the right side of the pig

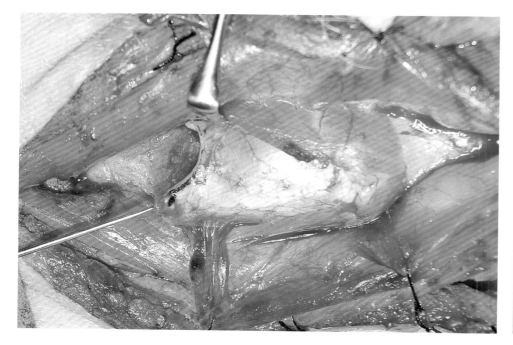

View of defect created by resecting thyroid ala graft and appearance of the graft once removed

Ruler is in cm gradations

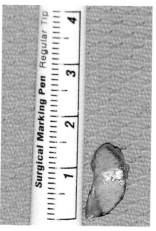

6

Anterior Laryngotracheoplasty Using Thyroid Ala Cartilage Graft (Single Stage)

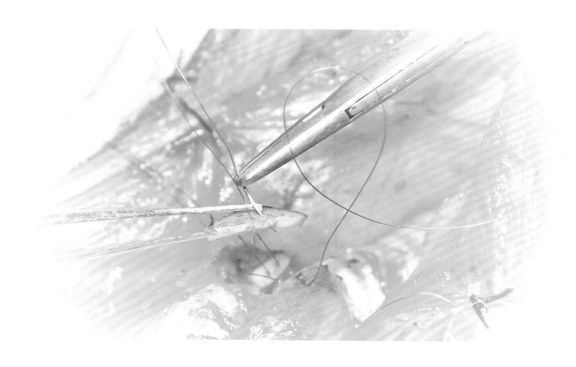

Disposable Items You Will Need

MEDICATIONS

- Akmezine
- Normal saline bag (3)

SHARPS

- 16- or 18-Gauge angiocatheter (1)
- 25-Gauge Butterfly needle (1)
- 2-0 Silk suture (7)
- 3-0 Polyglactin (Vicryl) suture on RB-1 tapered needle (3)
- 4-0 or 5-0 Polydioxanone (PDS) OR Polypropylene (Prolene) suture on RB-1 tapered needle (8)
- 4-0 Poliglecaprone (Monocryl) suture on P-3 reverse cutting needle (1)
- #15 blade (1)

OTHER

- 10 mL syringe (1)
- Intravenous tubing (1)
- 6.0 or 6.5 Cuffed endotracheal tube (1)
- Gloves (2 pairs)
- Strip of material (30 cm)
- Absorbent pad (1)
- Rope (180 cm)
- Marking pen (1)
- Ruler (1)
- Green towel (4)
- Penrose drain (1)

OPTIONAL

- None

Follow the steps outlined in "Exposure and Anatomy of the Pig Airway: Comparison with the Human Airway," "Anterior Cricoid Split," and "Harvest of Thyroid Ala Cartilage Graft" prior to performing this procedure.

Step 1 Place the thyroid ala graft into the defect created by the anterior cricoid split to confirm that its size and shape are appropriate. *In the pig, you may need to retract the thyroid cartilage superiorly with a cricoid hook to elongate the overlapping cartilages.*

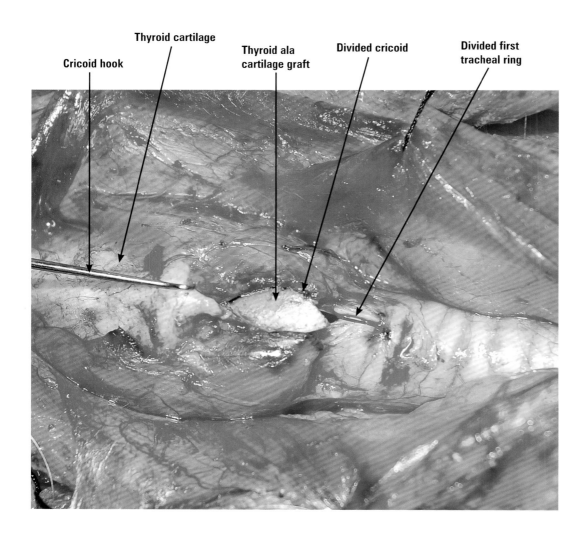

Cricoid hook   Thyroid cartilage   Thyroid ala cartilage graft   Divided cricoid   Divided first tracheal ring

Step 2 Suture the graft into the defect using either 4-0 or 5-0 sutures made of polydioxanone (PDS) or Prolene on a tapered needle. The benefit of the 4-0 suture is that it is less likely to break. The benefits of the PDS suture are that it has a bit of stretch to it that decreases the likelihood it will break when tying knots, and that it eventually resorbs after several months. The graft can be sutured with horizontal mattress sutures or simple interrupted sutures. We describe here the horizontal mattress suture technique.

A. Place the first suture from outside to inside through the tracheal cartilage.
B. Pass the needle through the lateral edge of the graft.
C. Come out through the anterior aspect of the graft.
D. Reenter the anterior aspect of the graft and exit through the lateral edge of the graft.
E. Reenter the edge of the tracheal cartilage and exit on the lateral surface. Five or six knots are tied on the lateral aspect of the trachea.

Horizontal Mattress Suture

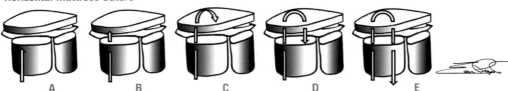

A   B   C   D   E

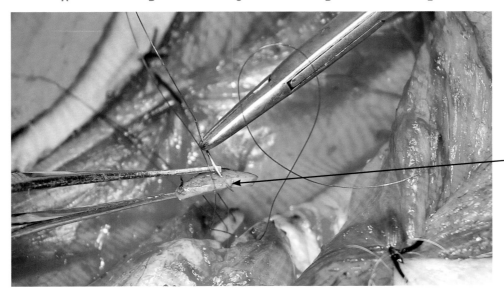

Suture being passed from anterior aspect of graft out through lateral edge of graft

Proponents of horizontal mattress sutures believe that placing the suture knots laterally allows for the strap muscles to directly contact the new graft anteriorly for better revascularization. If you do not believe this theory, then you may use simple interrupted sutures to suture the graft in place.

Try to minimize the number of needle passes through the cartilage because each needle pass injures chondrocytes in the graft. Each suture is pulled through until the two suture ends are even and a snap is placed to keep them together (tying the knots as you go makes it difficult to place additional sutures).

Step 3 Place sutures on both sides of the graft as well as superiorly and inferiorly to prevent an air leak. It is more important to prevent an air leak in single stage procedures. In double stage procedures, the air is more likely to leak around the tracheotomy tube than above it through a gap in the reconstructed airway.

Step 4 Arrange the "snapped" ends of the sutures neatly from superiorly to inferiorly. As one surgeon tightens each set of sutures from superiorly to inferiorly, the other surgeon allows the graft to "parachute" down into the defect. Tie the sutures with five to six knots.

Place sutures laterally, superiorly, and inferiorly

Parachute the graft down

Tie each suture pair with 5 to 6 knots

Check for air leak

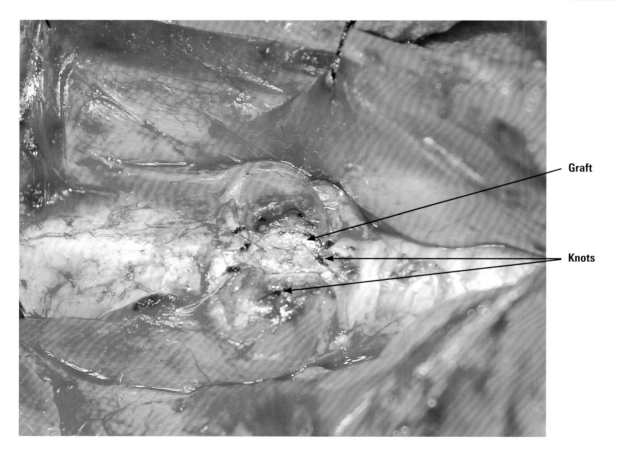

Graft

Knots

Step 5 Fill the wound with saline and perform a Valsalva maneuver to check for an air leak (demonstrated by bubbles in the saline). If a leak is present, additional simple interrupted sutures can be placed. *In humans, tissue glue can be used around the edges of the wound. However, we do not recommend wasting tissue glue while practicing on this porcine model. If there is no leak, suture the muscles closed using 3-0 Vicryl sutures and the skin with a 4-0 running Monocryl suture. Suture a Penrose drain in the lateral corner of the wound with a 2-0 silk suture.*

7

Harvest of Costal Cartilage Graft

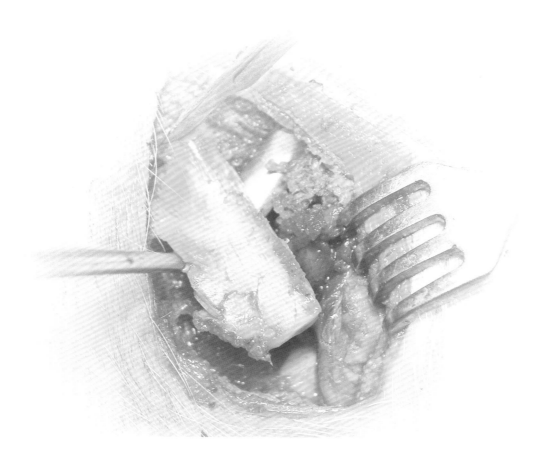

Disposable Items You Will Need

MEDICATIONS

- Akmezine
- Normal saline bag (3)

SHARPS

- 16- or 18-Gauge angiocatheter (1)
- 25-Gauge Butterfly needle (1)
- 27-Gauge angiocatheter (1)
- 2-0 Silk suture (5)
- 3-0 Polyglactin (Vicryl) suture (2)
- 4-0 Poliglecaprone (Monocryl) suture on P-3 reverse cutting needle (1)
- #15 Blade (1)

OTHER

- 10 mL syringe (1)
- Intravenous tubing (1)
- 6.0 or 6.5 Cuffed endotracheal tube (1)
- Gloves (2 pairs)
- Strip of material (30 cm)
- Absorbent pad (1)
- Rope (180 cm)
- Marking pen (1)
- Ruler (1)
- Green towel (4)
- Penrose drain (1)

OPTIONAL

- None

There are many differences between the rib cage of the pig and that of a human:

1. The sternum is much more narrow superiorly and flares to be much wider inferiorly as compared to that of a human.
2. The ribs attach to the sternum at a 45-degree angle rather than more perpendicularly, as seen in humans.
3. Each rib is thinner on its superior edge compared with that of a human rib making it more difficult to harvest.
4. The pig has an articulating joint laterally at the osteocartilaginous junction, whereas humans do not.

Pig ribs

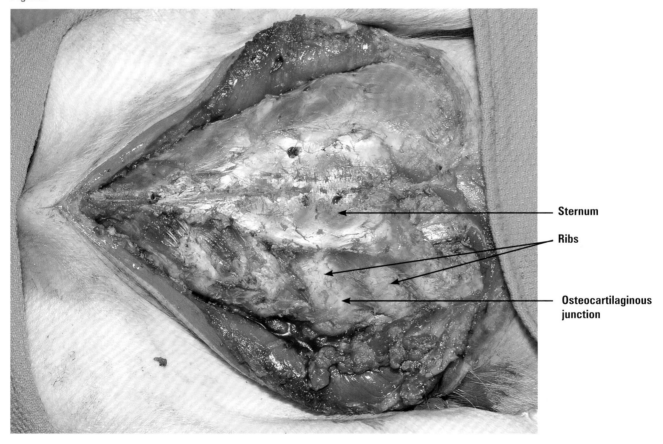

Sternum

Ribs

Osteocartilaginous junction

Prior to harvesting a rib in a human, ensure that the patient does not have a ventriculoperitoneal shunt. Along their path from the brain to the abdomen, these may course anterior to the ribs and deep to the chest wall musculature. Inadvertent injury of a ventriculoperitoneal shunt requires that it be replaced.

Harvest of Costal Cartilage Graft

Step 1 Mark a horizontal incision on the chest starting 1 cm lateral to the right lateral border of the sternum and extending laterally 4 cm. *Because the ribs slant infero-laterally in the pig, the incision may need to slant to reflect this variance. In human females, it is wise to place the chest incision in the location that will later become the infra mammary crease. To do this, gently pull up on the right nipple to create a skin crease. Mark the incision along this crease.*

KEY POINTS
Mark a horizontal incision 1 cm from sternal border and 4 cm long

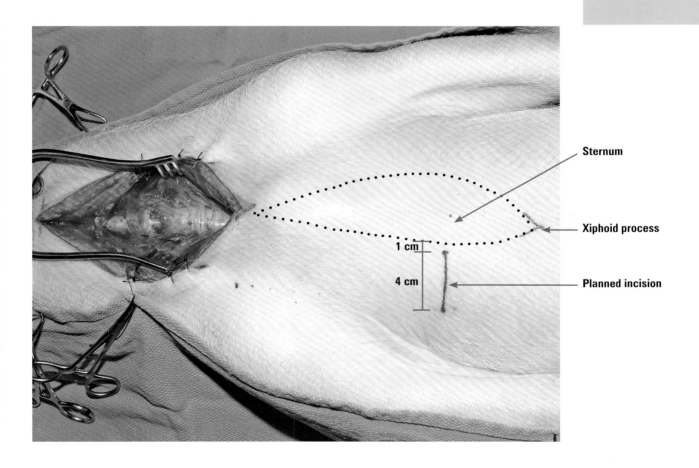

Step 2 Use a scalpel to incise through the skin. Use a microbipolar cautery to divide the muscle until you come down on to the costal cartilage. Try not to cauterize directly onto the cartilage because this could injure chondrocytes and decrease the viability of the graft. The wound can be retracted open by your assistant holding two Seine retractors, a self-retaining retractor, or 2-0 silk sutures.

Costal cartilage   Seine rake

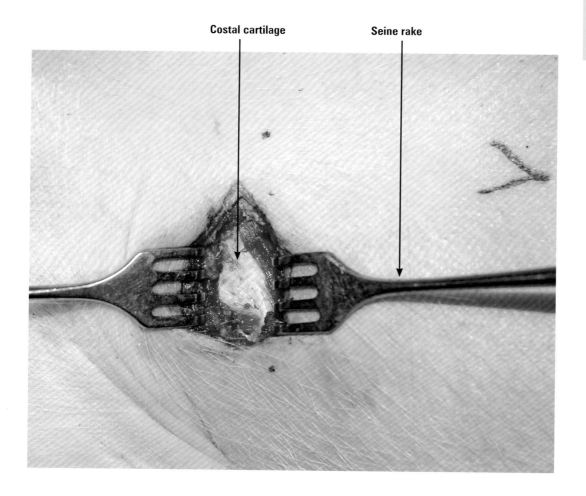

Step 3 *In humans, it is equally as easy to elevate the perichondrium off the superior and inferior edges of the costal cartilage. However, in the sus scrofa piglet, the superior border is very thin and the inferior border is thick like in humans. We therefore suggest elevating the perichondrium off the inferior border first to get accustomed to the surgery.*

Step 4 Stand on the right side of the pig at the foot of the bed and face its head. Use a skin hook to retract the inferior edge of the rib anteriorly.

Step 5 With a suction in your left hand and a #15 scalpel in your right hand, gently incise the perichondrium. Try not to cut too deeply into the rib itself as this will compromise the quality of the flanges you will later be carving.

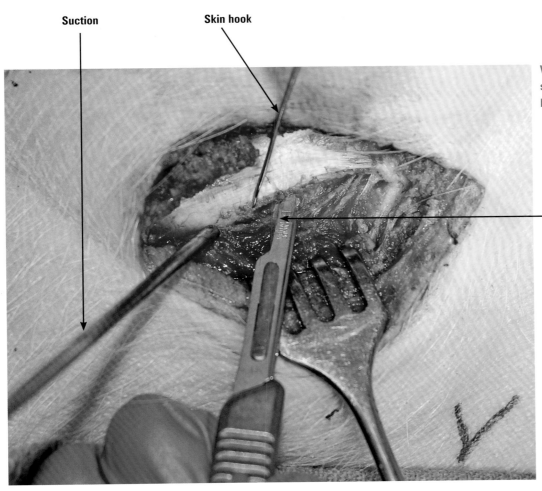

Suction

Skin hook

View while standing on the right side of the pig at the foot of the bed facing the head of the pig

Scalpel

Step 6 Use a Freer elevator to elevate the posterior perichondrium off the inferior half of the rib. This dissection is carried superiorly halfway up the posterior side of the rib. The angle of dissection makes it difficult to elevate the perichondrium off the entire rib. Attempting to do this may cause you to inadvertently puncture through the perichondrium and cause a pneumothorax. For this reason, the superior half of the posterior perichondrium is elevated off the rib through a separate superior incision.

KEY POINTS
Elevate posterior perichondrium from inferiorly

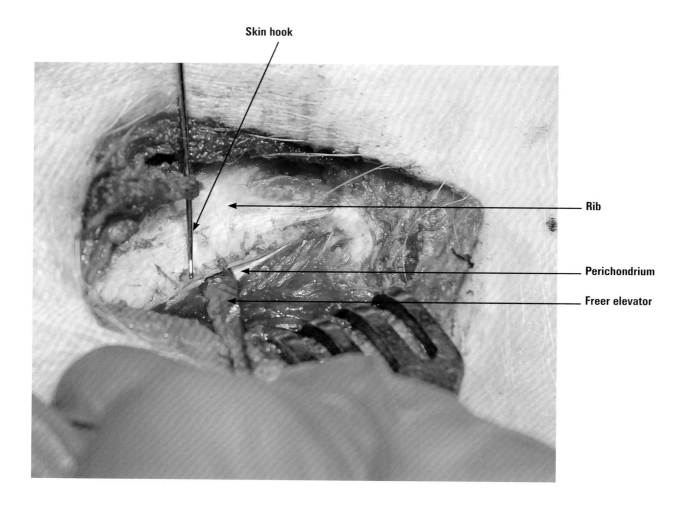

Skin hook

Rib

Perichondrium

Freer elevator

Step 7 Stand on the right side of the pig at the head of the bed and face its feet. With a suction in your left hand and a scalpel in your right hand, incise the perichondrium along the superior edge of the rib.

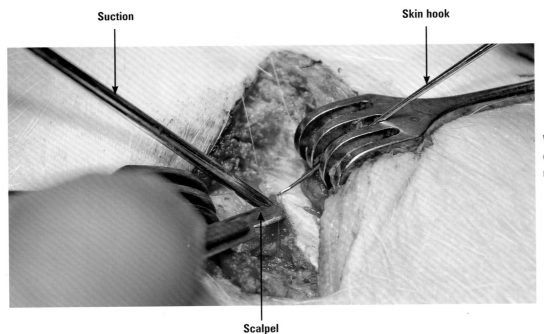

Suction

Skin hook

Scalpel

View while standing on right side of pig at head of bed looking inferiorly facing the pig's feet

Step 8 Use a Freer elevator to elevate the posterior perichondrium off the superior half of the rib. *As mentioned previously, the superior edge of the rib in the sus scrofa piglet is much thinner than in humans, making elevation of the perichondrium along the superior edge more difficult.*

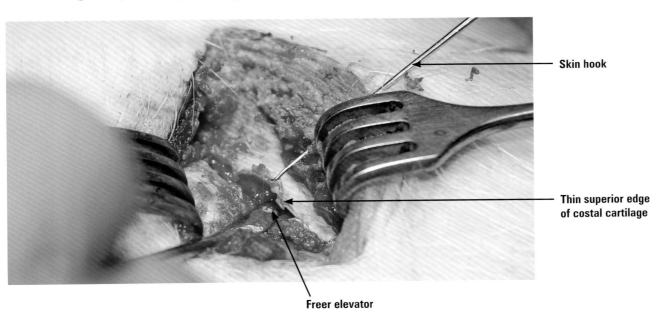

Skin hook

Thin superior edge of costal cartilage

Freer elevator

Step 9 When the Freer elevator can pass through both sides and the two tissue planes are joined, slide the Freer medially and laterally to elevate the remaining perichondrium off the posterior aspect of the rib. The medial limit is the perichondrial attachment to the sternum and the lateral limit is the perichondrial attachment to the osseocartilaginous junction. If you are having difficulty elevating the perichondrium off the cartilage, you are likely working too close to the osseocartilaginous junction and you should try working more medially.

KEY POINTS

Join superior and inferior dissection planes

Slide Freer elevator medially and laterally

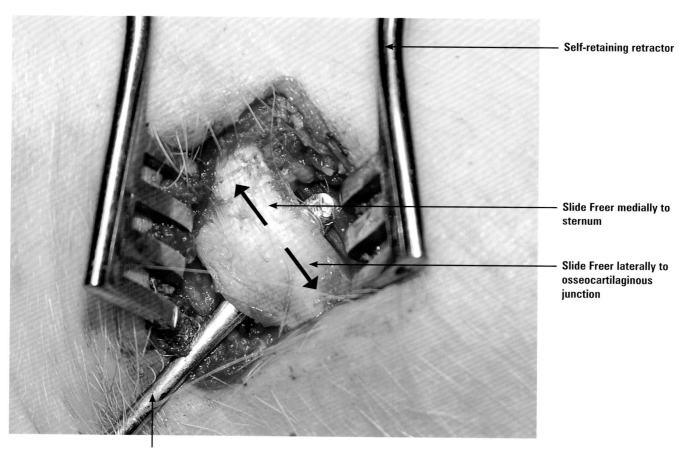

Self-retaining retractor

Slide Freer medially to sternum

Slide Freer laterally to osseocartilaginous junction

Freer elevator

Step 10 Place the back end of a Seine retractor deep to the rib, as shown, to protect the perichondrium and the lung when dividing the rib. To delineate the exact border between the osseous rib and the cartilaginous rib (osseocartilaginous junction), gently poke a small needle (i.e., 27-g) through the rib and see how easily it passes through. The needle will pass through cartilage much more easily than it will through bone. To avoid passing through the rib and puncturing the pleura of the lung, place a snap on the shaft of the needle 5 mm away from its tip. Use a #15 blade to cut through the cartilaginous side of the junction. Cut down onto the back end of the metal Seine retractor to prevent puncturing the pleura of the lung.

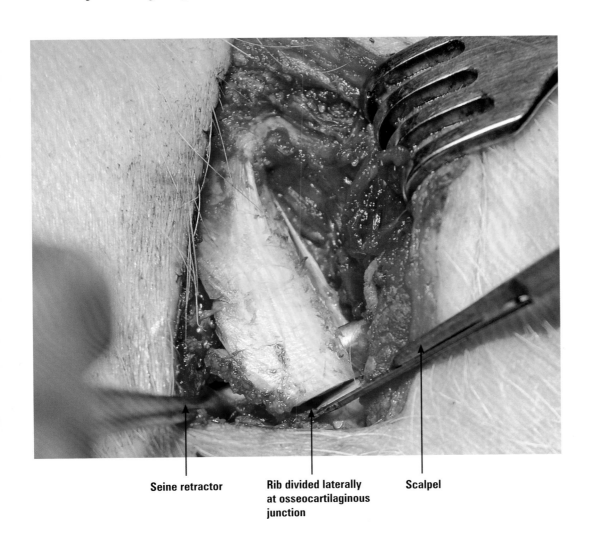

Seine retractor   **Rib divided laterally at osseocartilaginous junction**   **Scalpel**

Step 11 Slide the back end of the Seine retractor medially to ensure the perichondrium is elevated as far medially as possible. You may also have your assistant retract the cut lateral end of the rib anteriorly while you visualize its posterior edge and elevate the remaining perichondrium off the rib medially using a Freer elevator.

Seine retractor sliding medially

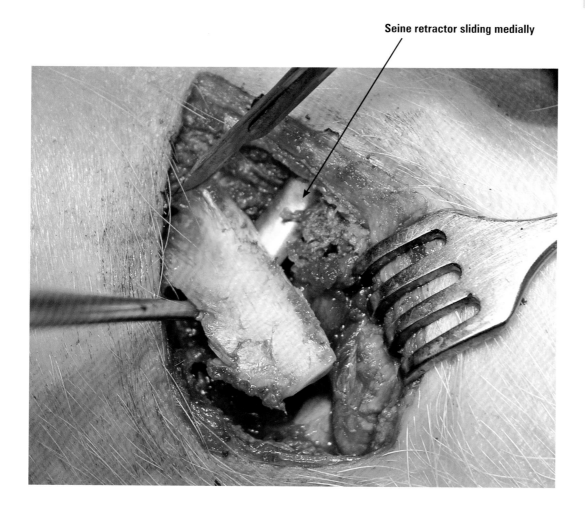

Step 12 When you have elevated the rib off the perichondrium medially to the sternum, measure the length of rib that you are about to harvest. If it is long enough to fit into the cricoid split defect you created (see Chapter 4), place the back end of your Seine retractor against the posterior edge of the rib and cut down onto it, dividing the rib along its medial aspect. *In humans, if the rib is not long enough to fit into the cricoid split defect, you may either lengthen the rib by cutting into the sternum (not possible in piglets due to the thin sternum), or you may harvest a second rib.*

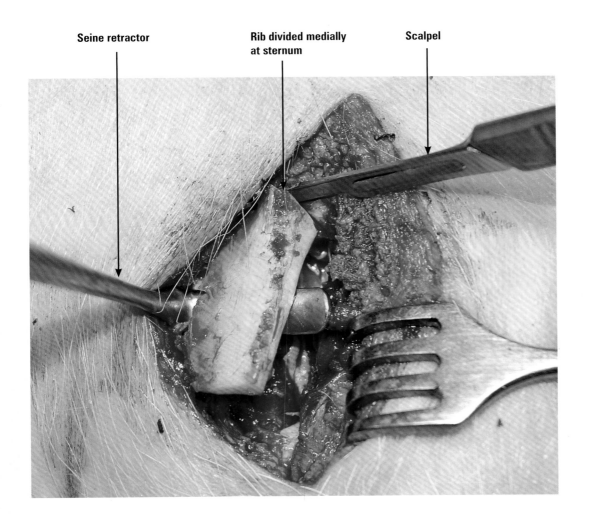

Seine retractor

Rib divided medially at sternum

Scalpel

Step 13 Remove the rib and irrigate the wound. Fill the wound with sterile saline and perform a Valsalva maneuver while looking for air bubbles that would signify a tear in the pleura. If there is no leak, suture the muscles closed using 3-0 Vicryl sutures and the skin with a running Monocryl suture. Suture a Penrose drain in the lateral corner of the wound with a 2-0 silk suture to allow any collected fluid or air to drain out.

KEY POINTS

Irrigate wound

Valsalva to check for pleural leak

Close wound with Vicryl and Monocryl sutures

Rib Anterior Surface

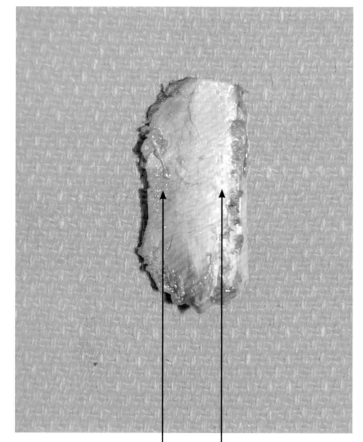

Thin superior edge   Thick inferior edge

Rib Posterior Surface

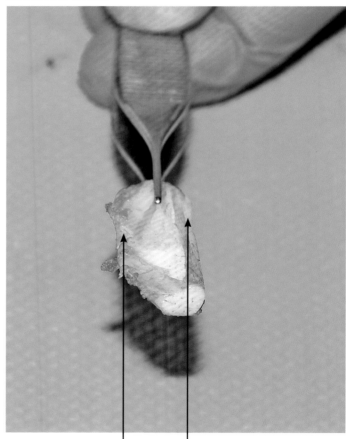

Thin superior edge   Thick inferior edge

8

Anterior Laryngotracheoplasty Using Costal Cartilage Graft (Single Stage)

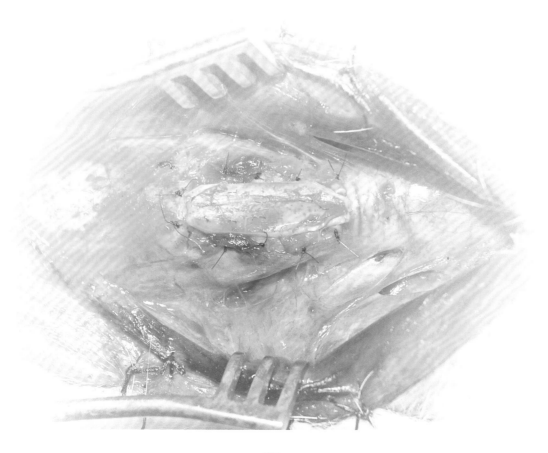

Disposable Items You Will Need

MEDICATIONS

- Akmezine
- Normal saline bag (3)

SHARPS

- 16- or 18-Gauge angiocatheter (1)
- 25-Gauge Butterfly needle (1)
- 27-Gauge angiocatheter (1)
- 2-0 Silk suture (7)
- 3-0 Polyglactin (Vicryl) suture (5)
- 4-0 or 5-0 Polydioxanone (PDS)
  OR Polypropylene (Prolene) suture on
  RB-1 tapered needle (8)
- 4-0 Poliglecaprone (Monocryl) suture on
  P-3 reverse cutting needle (2)
- #15 Blade (1)
- #10 Blade (1)

OTHER

- 10 mL syringe (1)
- Intravenous tubing (1)
- 6.0 or 6.5 Cuffed endotracheal tube (1)
- Gloves (2 pairs)
- Strip of material (30 cm)
- Absorbent pad (1)
- Rope (180 cm)
- Marking pen (1)
- Ruler (1)
- Green towel (8)
- Penrose drain (2)

OPTIONAL

- None

Anterior Laryngotracheoplasty Using Costal Cartilage Graft (Single Stage)

Follow the steps outlined in "Exposure and Anatomy of the Pig Airway: Comparison with the Human Airway," "Anterior Cricoid Split," and "Harvest of Costal Cartilage Graft" prior to performing this procedure.

Step 1 Extend the anterior cricoid split inferiorly by dividing an additional one to two tracheal rings inferiorly in the midline. This will allow you to practice suturing a graft into a larger defect.

KEY POINTS

Extend the anterior cricoid split inferiorly

Measure the length of the defect

Anterior Cricoid Split

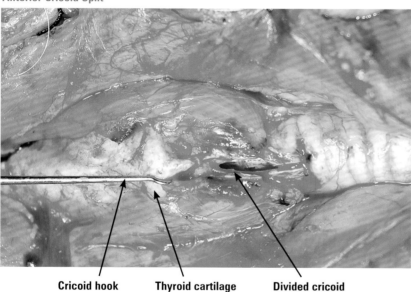

Cricoid hook   Thyroid cartilage   Divided cricoid

Extended Anterior Cricoid Split

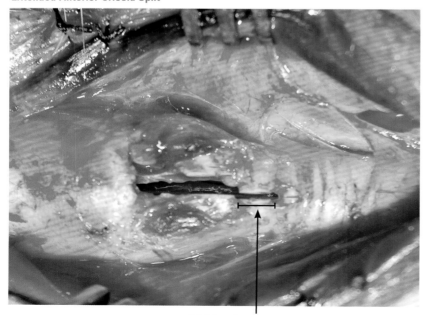

Additional tracheal rings divided

KEY POINTS

Cut off thin edge of
graft in pig

Step 2 Use a caliper or ruler to measure the length of the defect and write this number down.

Step 3 *The rib in the pig is much thinner superiorly than it is in humans.* Cut off the thin superior edge of the graft to make it easier to carve flanges.

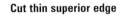

Cut thin superior edge

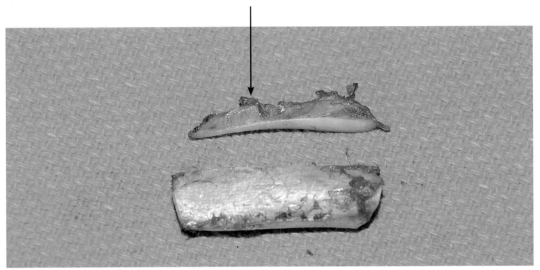

Anterior Laryngotracheoplasty Using Costal Cartilage Graft (Single Stage)

Step 4 Use a marking pen to draw an ellipse on the anterior surface of the graft that still has perichondrium on it. The length should match the measured length of the extended anterior cricoid split. The width should be as large as possible while allowing flanges to be carved, which in the pig is approximately 4 to 5 mm *(5–6 mm in humans)*. The flanges around the edges will be approximately 2 mm wide. Draw a line on the side of the graft denoting half the thickness of the graft.

KEY POINTS

Draw ellipse

Balance between large width for maximal distraction and wide flanges

Draw line denoting half the thickness

Incise along side of graft

Incise around ellipse

Anterior Surface of Rib Graft

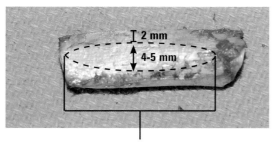

2 mm

4-5 mm

Length of extended anterior cricoid split

Side of Rib Graft

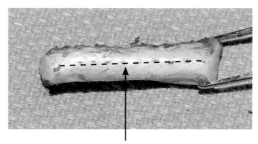

Line denoting half of the thickness

Step 5 Use a #10 scalpel to incise along the line denoting half the thickness of the graft to a depth of 2 mm. Repeat on the other side of the rib graft. Incise along the marked ellipse on the anterior surface of the rib graft down to the level of the lateral cuts.

Amount of distraction   Width of flange

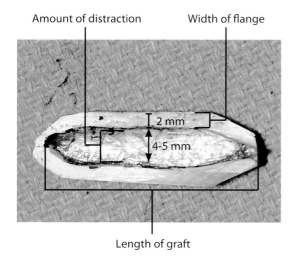

2 mm

4-5 mm

Length of graft

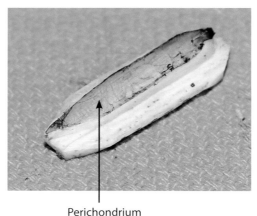

Perichondrium

Anterior Laryngotracheoplasty Using Costal Cartilage Graft (Single Stage)

8

Step 6 Suture the graft into the defect using either 4-0 or 5-0 sutures made of polydioxanone (PDS) or Prolene. The benefit of the 4-0 suture is that it is less likely to break. Benefits of the PDS suture are that it has a bit of stretch to it that decreases the likelihood it will break when tying knots, and that it eventually resorbs after several months. The graft can be sutured with horizontal mattress sutures or simple interrupted sutures. We describe here the horizontal mattress suture technique.

A. Pass the needle through the tracheal cartilage from outside to inside, coming out submucosally on the lumenal side.
B. Pass the suture through the right angle formed by the flange and the graft.
C. Exit through the midline of the graft.
D. Pass the suture back through the graft and exit through the right angle formed by the flange and the graft.
E. Enter the tracheal cartilage submucosally passing from medial to lateral.

Snap the suture ends together. Try to make these suture ends equal in length by adjusting the suture length after each pass through cartilage rather than after passing through all of the cartilages. Pulling the suture through after passing through all cartilages risks tearing the cartilage.

KEY POINTS

Suture the graft using 4-0 or 5-0 sutures

Horizontal mattress or simple interrupted sutures

Sutures pass through lumenal side submucosally

Sutures pass through right angle formed by graft and flange

Pull suture through after each pass through cartilage

Horizontal Mattress Sutures

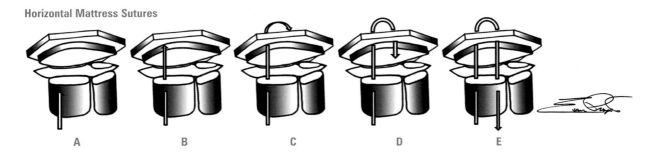

A   B   C   D   E

Proponents of horizontal mattress sutures believe that placing the suture knots laterally allows for the strap muscles to directly contact the new graft anteriorly for better revascularization. If you do not believe this theory, then you may use simple interrupted sutures to suture the graft in place.

Try to minimize the number of needle passes through the cartilage because each needle pass injures the chondrocytes in the graft. Each suture is pulled through until the two suture ends are even and a snap is placed to keep them together (tying the knots as you go makes it difficult to place additional sutures).

Anterior Laryngotracheoplasty Using Costal Cartilage Graft (Single Stage)

8

Step 7 Place sutures along both sides of the graft as well as superiorly and inferiorly to prevent an air leak. It is important to prevent an air leak in single-stage procedures. In double-stage procedures, the air is more likely to leak around the tracheotomy tube than above it through a gap in the reconstructed airway.

Step 8 Arrange the "snapped" ends of the sutures neatly from superiorly to inferiorly. As one surgeon tightens each set of sutures from superiorly to inferiorly, the other surgeon allows the graft to "parachute" down into the defect. Tie the sutures with five to six knots.

KEY POINTS

Place sutures laterally, superiorly and inferiorly

Parachute the graft down and tie each suture pair with 5 to 6 knots

Check for air leak

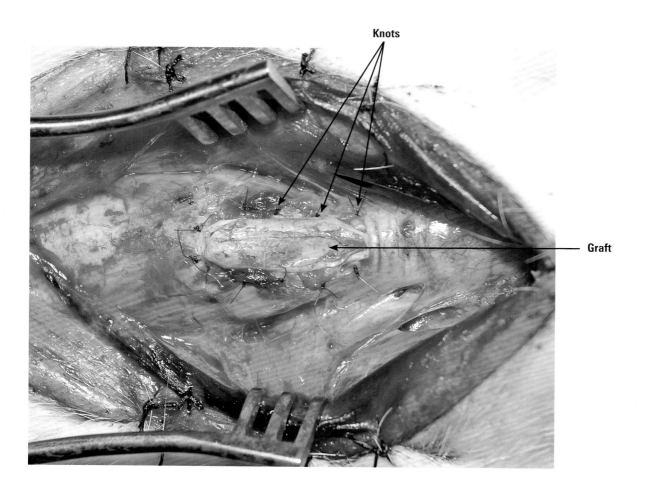

Knots

Graft

Step 9 Fill the wound with saline and perform a Valsalva maneuver to check for an air leak (demonstrated by bubbles in the saline). If a leak is present, additional simple interrupted sutures can be placed. *In humans, tissue glue can be used around the edges of the wound. However, we do not recommend wasting tissue glue while practicing on this porcine model.* If there is no leak, suture the muscles closed using 3-0 Vicryl sutures and the skin with a 4-0 running Monocryl suture. Suture a Penrose drain in the lateral corner of the wound with a 2-0 silk suture.

9

Posterior Laryngotracheoplasty Using Costal Cartilage Graft (Single Stage)

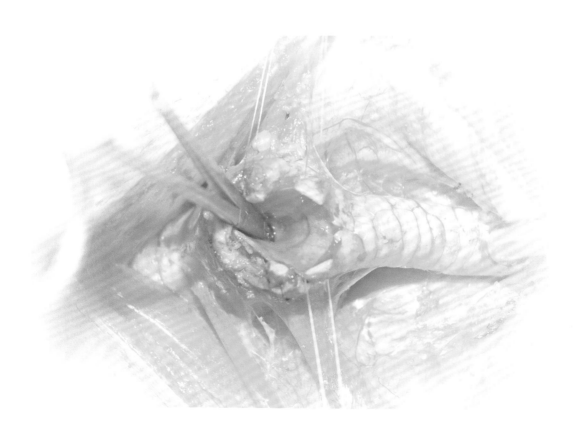

Disposable Items You Will Need

MEDICATIONS

- Akmezine
- Lidocaine 1% with 1/100,000 Epinephrine
- Pledget with oxymetazoline
  OR topical epinephrine (4)
- Normal saline bag (3)

SHARPS

- 16- or 18-Gauge angiocatheter (1)
- 25-Gauge Butterfly needle (1)
- 25-Gauge angiocatheter (1)
- 27-Gauge angiocatheter (1)
- 2-0 Silk suture (9)
- 3-0 Polyglactin (Vicryl) suture (5)
- 4-0 Polypropylene (Prolene) suture on
  RB-1 tapered needle (4)
- 4-0 or 5-0 Polydioxanone (PDS)
  OR Polypropylene (Prolene) suture on
  RB-1 tapered needle (4)
- 4-0 Poliglecaprone (Monocryl) suture on
  P-3 reverse cutting needle (2)
- #15 Blade (1)
- #10 Blade (1)
- Beaver blade (1)

OTHER

- 10 mL syringe (2)
- Intravenous tubing (1)
- 6.0 or 6.5 Cuffed endotracheal tube (1)
- Second endotracheal tube (cuffed
  6.5 armored OR 7.0 oral RAE
  OR regular cuffed 6.5)
- Gloves (2 pairs)
- Strip of material (30 cm)
- Absorbent pad (1)
- Rope (180 cm)
- Marking pen (1)
- Ruler (1)
- Green towel (8)
- Penrose drain (2)

OPTIONAL

- Red rubber catheter (1)

Posterior Laryngotracheoplasty Using Costal Cartilage Graft (Single Stage)

Follow the steps outlined in *"Exposure and Anatomy of the Pig Airway: Comparison with the Human Airway."*

Step 1 Perform a temporary tracheotomy so the posterior cricoid plate can be visualized without being obscured by the endotracheal tube. An armored endotracheal tube with the cuff deflated works well for this. You may also use a modified RAE tube as demonstrated in "Placing a Stent" on page 94. However, a regular endotracheal tube will suffice if costs are a consideration. Suture the endotracheal tube to the chest with 2-0 silk sutures, and place it off to the left side of the chest.

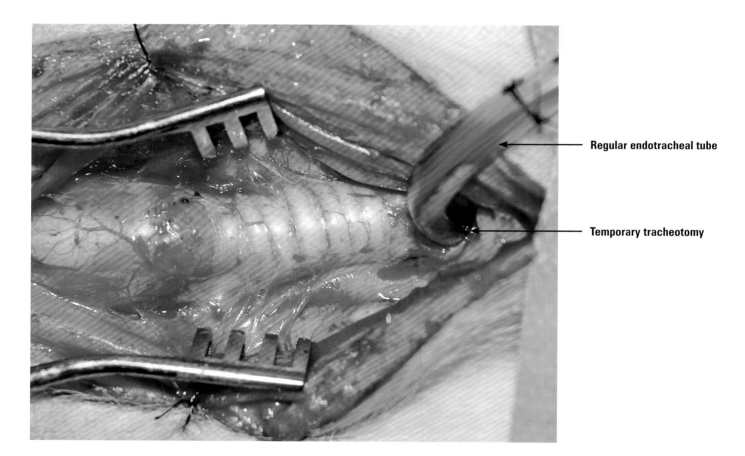

KEY POINTS
Temporary tracheotomy

Regular endotracheal tube

Temporary tracheotomy

Step 2 Follow the steps outlined in *"Anterior Cricoid Split"* and *"Harvest of Costal Cartilage Graft"* prior to performing this procedure.

Step 3 Extend the anterior cricoid split inferiorly by dividing an additional one to two tracheal rings. This will allow you to see the posterior cricoid plate clearly.

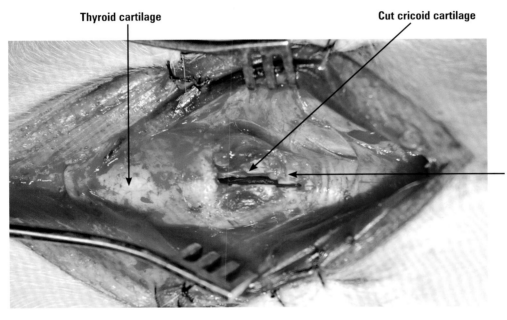

Thyroid cartilage   Cut cricoid cartilage

Extended anterior cricoid split

Step 4 Place a 4-0 Prolene retraction suture through each side of the split cricoid to retract it open. You may need to place retraction sutures through the divided tracheal rings if you require better exposure.

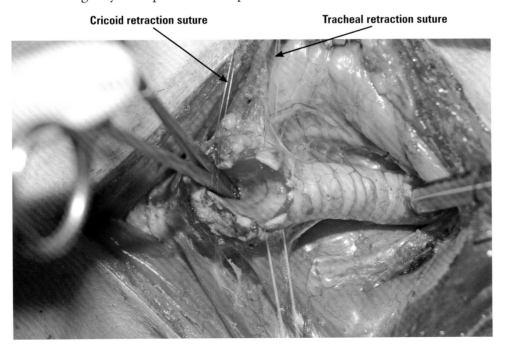

Cricoid retraction suture   Tracheal retraction suture

Step 5 Place a Lauer (Mixter/right-angled snap) over the superior edge of the posterior cricoid plate with the tips facing inferiorly into the esophagus. This brings the posterior cricoid plate inferiorly so you can divide it without having to perform a laryngofissure.

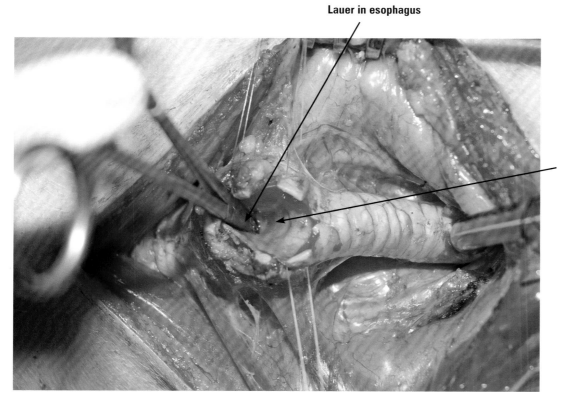

Lauer in esophagus

Posterior cricoid plate

Step 6 Infiltrate the mucosa overlying the posterior cricoid plate with lidocaine with epinephrine and then pass the needle through the posterior cricoid plate to infiltrate the space immediately posterior to it for hemostasis and hydrodissection. Place a pledget with oxymetazoline or topical epinephrine directly on the mucosa of the posterior cricoid plate for additional hemostasis.

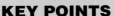
Step 7 Use a straight beaver blade to divide the posterior cricoid plate vertically in the midline. The posterior cricoid plate is usually thicker (anteroposterior dimension) and taller (craniocaudal dimension) than anticipated in both humans and pigs. *In humans, you will also need to divide the interarytenoid muscle to prevent arytenoid prolapse. However, this is difficult to do in pigs and may be omitted here.*

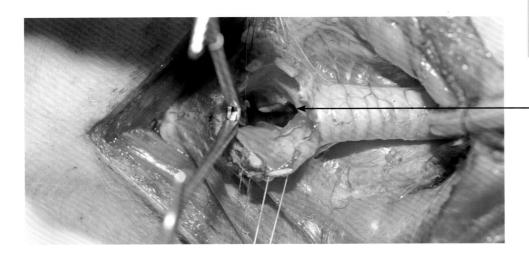

Cut edge of divided posterior cricoid plate

Step 8 Use a Freer elevator or a round knife to elevate the muscle off the posterior aspect of the posterior cricoid plate. This creates two lateral pockets into which the flanges of the posterior graft can snap snuggly. Be careful not to perforate through the muscle into the postcricoid esophagus.

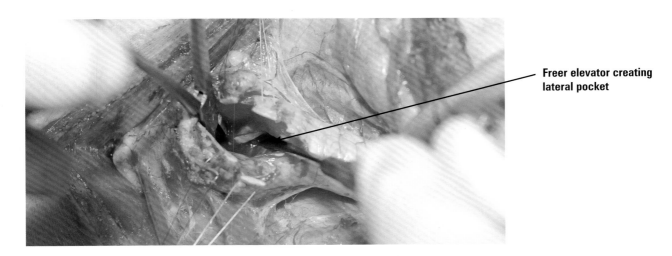

Freer elevator creating lateral pocket

Step 9 *The rib in the pig is much thinner superiorly than it is in humans.* Cut off the thin superior edge of the graft to make it easier to carve flanges.

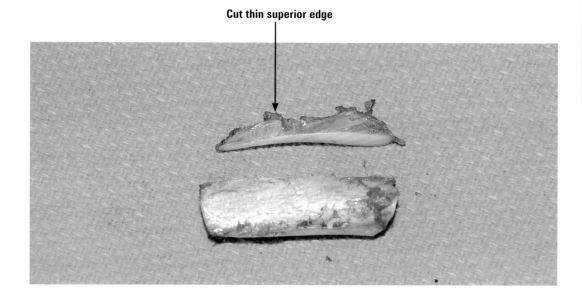

Cut thin superior edge

Step 10 Use a marking pen to draw a rectangle on the anterior surface of the graft that still has perichondrium on it. The length should be long enough to extend from the arytenoids to the inferior border of the posterior cricoid plate, but is often shorter than this. The width should be approximately 4 to 5 mm, because making the graft wider than this may cause aspiration. Draw a line on the side of the graft denoting half the thickness of the graft.

Anterior Surface of Rib Graft

Side of Rib Graft

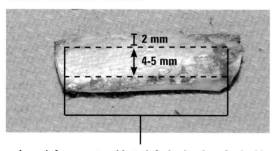

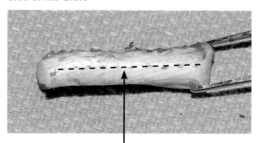

2 mm

4-5 mm

Length from arytenoids to inferior border of cricoid

Line denoting half of the thickness

11

Tracheotomy

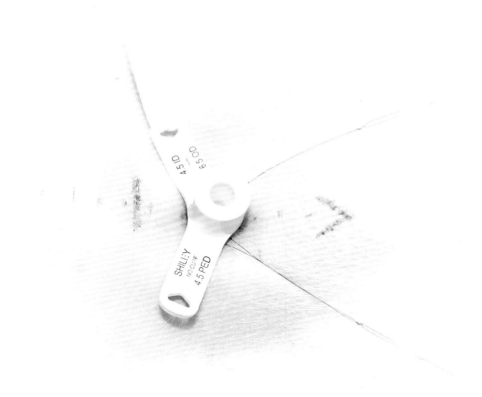

Disposable Items You Will Need

MEDICATIONS

- Akmezine
- Lidocaine 1% with 1/100,000 Epinephrine
- Pledget with oxymetazoline or topical epinephrine (1)
- Normal saline bag (3)

SHARPS

- 16- or 18-Gauge angiocatheter (1)
- 25-Gauge Butterfly needle (1)
- 4-0 Prolene suture on RB-1 tapered needle (2)
- 3-0 Chromic gut suture on SH-1 tapered needle (4)
- #15 Blade (1)

OTHER

- 10 mL syringe (1)
- Intravenous tubing (1)
- 6.0 or 6.5 Cuffed endotracheal tube (1)
- Gloves (2 pairs)
- Strip of material (30 cm)
- Absorbent pad (1)
- Rope (180 cm)
- Marking pen (1)
- Ruler (1)
- Green towel (4)
- Sterile adhesive strips (2)
- 4.5 PED tracheotomy with ties (1)

OPTIONAL

- None

Tracheotomy

Tracheotomy is a surgical method of obtaining a safe airway by bypassing an upper airway obstruction. Human patients may already have a tracheotomy if you are planning to perform an open laryngotracheoplasty. If they do not already have a tracheotomy and you are planning to perform a double-stage laryngotracheoplasty, you will have to perform a tracheotomy at the beginning of the open airway surgery. There are many ways to perform a tracheotomy, and the variations are too numerous to describe here. We therefore describe here one method that incorporates many of these techniques.

KEY POINTS

Draw a horizontal line at level of hyoid bone

Draw a horizontal line at level of cricoid cartilage

Mark sternal notch

Mark planned incision

Step 1 Draw a horizontal line at the level of the hyoid bone and another horizontal line at the level of the cricoid cartilage. Draw a ">" marking the sternal notch. Draw a horizontal line 2 cm long located 2 cm below the cricoid cartilage to mark the planned incision.

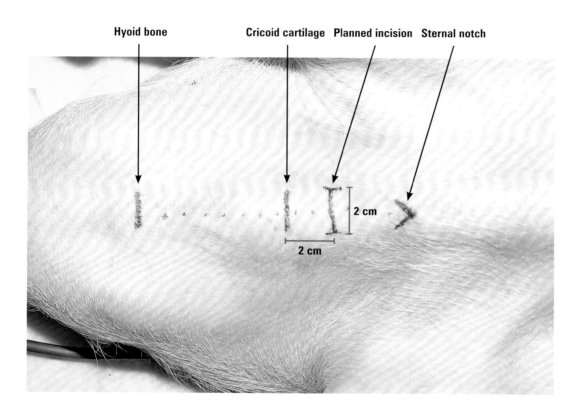

Hyoid bone   Cricoid cartilage   Planned incision   Sternal notch

2 cm

2 cm

Tracheotomy

Step 2 Incise the skin with a #15 blade and retract the soft tissue with Seine retractors.

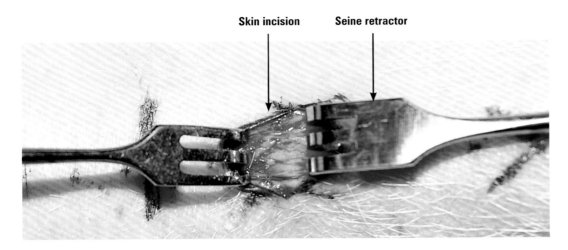

Skin incision   Seine retractor

Step 3 Remove the subcutaneous fat down to the level of the sternohyoid muscles using bipolar cautery.

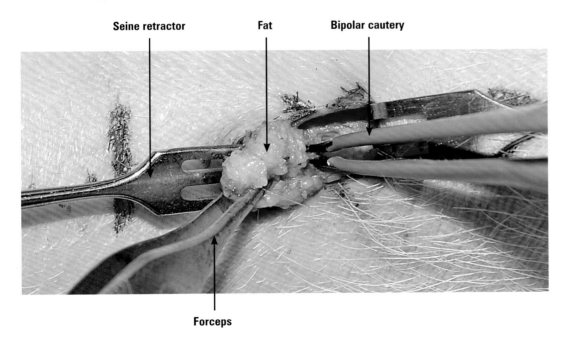

Seine retractor   Fat   Bipolar cautery

Forceps

Tracheotomy

11

Step 4 Retract each sternohyoid muscle laterally.

KEY POINTS

Retract sternohyoid muscles laterally

Divide sternohyoid muscles vertically

Left sternohyoid muscle

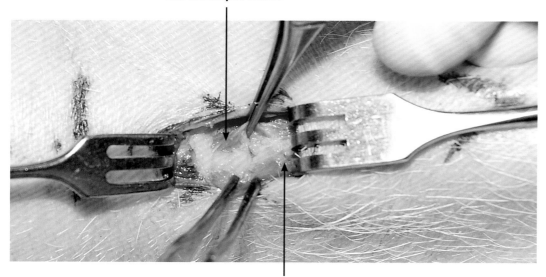

Right sternohyoid muscle

Step 5 Divide the sternohyoid muscles vertically in the midline.

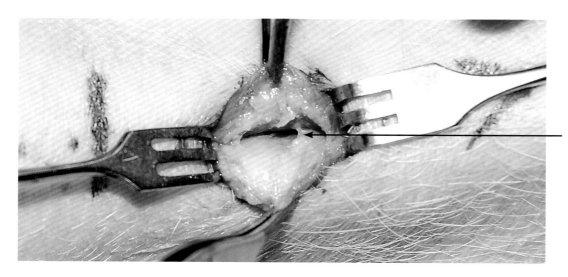

Sternohyoid muscles divided in midline

Airway Reconstruction Surgical Dissection Manual

79

Step 6 Retract the sternohyoid muscles laterally using Seine retractors or ribbon retractors.

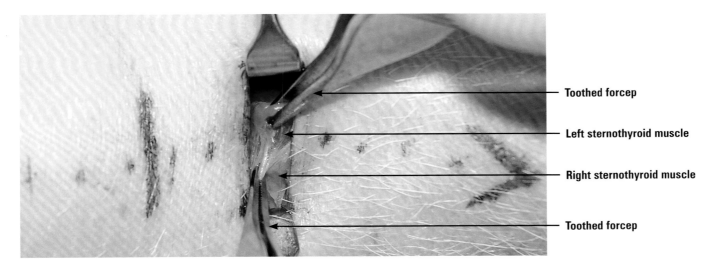

— Seine retractor

— Seine retractor

Step 7 Retract each sternothyroid muscle laterally.

— Toothed forcep

— Left sternothyroid muscle

— Right sternothyroid muscle

— Toothed forcep

Step 8 Divide the sternothyroid muscles vertically in the midline.

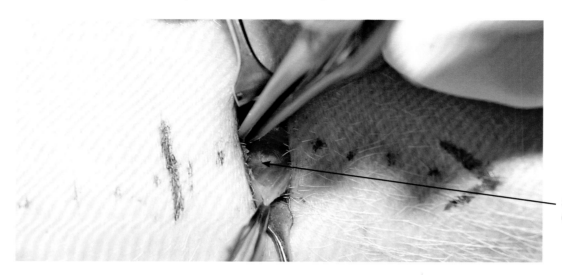

Sternothyroid muscles divided in midline

Step 9 Retract the sternothyroid muscles laterally to expose the underlying trachea. If you are unsure whether you are looking at the trachea (as can be the case in neonates or patients without cartilaginous rings such as in the case of a sleeve trachea), place a 27-gauge needle on a syringe filled with saline, poke this into the structure, and aspirate. If you see air bubbles then you are in the trachea. If you see blood then you are in a vessel.

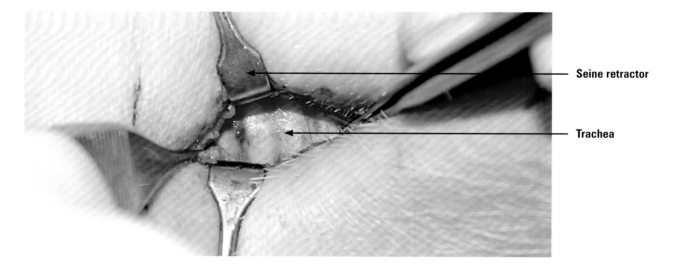

Seine retractor

Trachea

KEY POINTS

Cauterize trachea

Retract trachea anteriorly with cricoid hook

Incise trachea vertically

Cut through 2 or 3 tracheal rings

Step 10 Gently cauterize a vertical line on the trachea where you intend to make your tracheotomy. This will decrease the amount of bleeding when you make the incision. Place a cricoid hook in the inferior aspect of the cricoid cartilage to retract the trachea anteriorly and superiorly (to make it easier to enter) and provide stability.

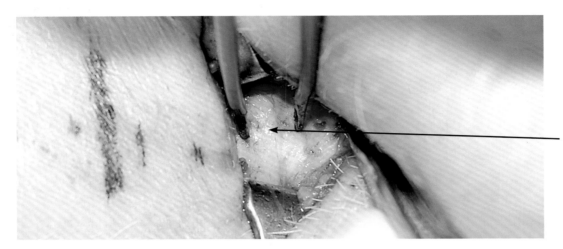

Cauterized line

Step 11 Ask the anesthesiologist to deflate the cuff on the endotracheal tube (if there is one) to avoid damaging it when you enter the airway. Incise the trachea with a #15 blade. Make your incision vertically in the midline from inferiorly to superiorly to decrease the possibility of injuring the innominate (brachiocephalic) artery. Cut through two or three tracheal rings. If blood begins to drip into the tracheotomy, place a pledget soaked in epinephrine or oxymetazoline into the tracheotomy. Do NOT use cautery after entering the trachea because it can lead to an airway fire.

Before Incision

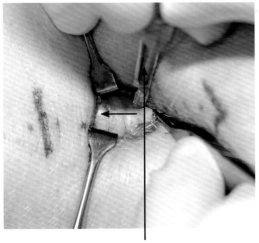

Scalpel

After Incision

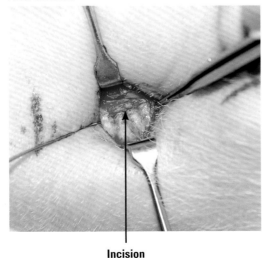

Incision

Step 12 **Stay Sutures.** Pass a 4-0 Prolene "stay suture" along the cut edges of two cartilaginous rings at the lateral edge of the tracheotomy. Place the suture from inferiorly to superiorly to avoid injuring the innominate (brachiocephalic) artery. Repeat on the other side of the tracheotomy incision. In the event that the tracheotomy accidentally falls out of the airway postoperatively, these sutures can be pulled laterally to open the airway in an emergency.

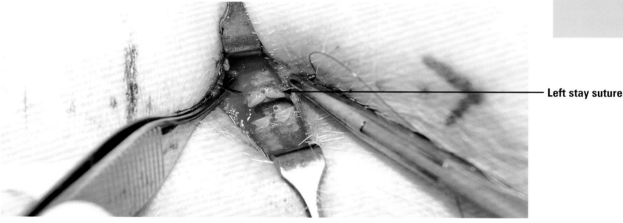

Left stay suture

Step 13 Tie two knots in each "stay suture" as shown. Place sterile adhesive strips marked "right" and "left" through the loops and tape each of these sutures to their respective side of the chest with clear adhesive tape. Pull these gently to open the tracheotomy.

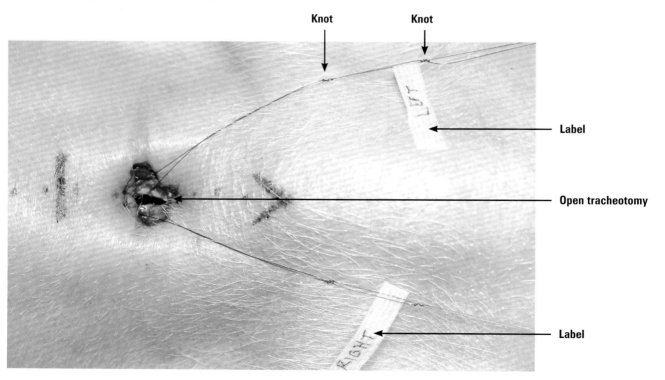

Knot   Knot

Label

Open tracheotomy

Label

Step 14 **Maturation Sutures.** Use 3-0 chromic sutures to "mature" the tracheotomy stoma. "Maturing" the stoma involves suturing the skin to the tracheal cartilage to hasten the natural process of tract formation. To do this, place two horizontal mattress sutures at the inferior edge and two horizontal mattress sutures at the superior edge of the tracheotomy. Place the inferior maturation sutures close together to prevent the tracheotomy tube from slipping into a false passage between the skin and the trachea.

A. Pass the suture through the skin.
B. Enter the trachea inferior to the inferior aspect of the tracheotomy. Exit the trachea through the tracheotomy stoma.
C. Pass the suture out through the skin.
D. Pull the suture through and hold both ends together with a snap.

KEY POINTS

Suture to "mature" tracheotomy stoma

A

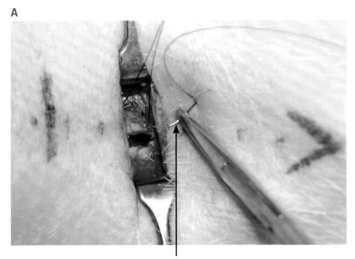

Suture through skin

B

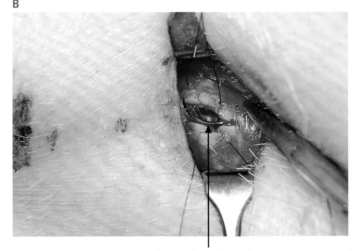

Suture through trachea

C

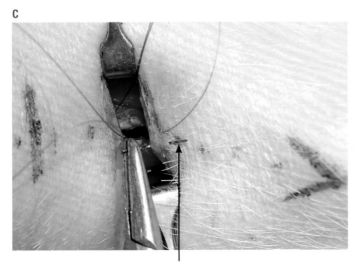

Suture back through skin

D

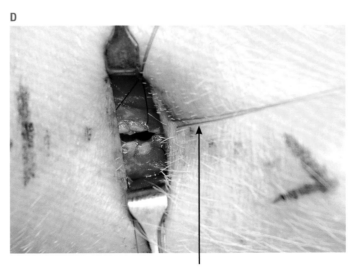

Both ends of suture through skin

Step 15 Place the three remaining sutures and tie each of the four sutures with multiple knots.

KEY POINTS

Place 3 remaining sutures

Tie the 4 sutures with multiple knots

Ask anesthesiologist to remove tape securing endotracheal tube from mouth and nose. Stop when distal tip reaches superior aspect of the tracheotomy stoma

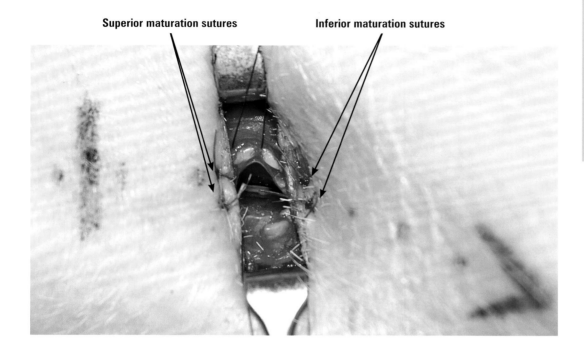

Superior maturation sutures   Inferior maturation sutures

Step 16 Ask the anesthesiologist to remove the tape securing the endotracheal tube from around the mouth or nose and withdraw it very slowly as you observe it moving superiorly while viewing it through the tracheotomy stoma. Tell the anesthesiologist to stop withdrawing when the distal tip of the endotracheal tube reaches the superior aspect of the tracheotomy stoma.

Before Withdrawal of Endotracheal Tube

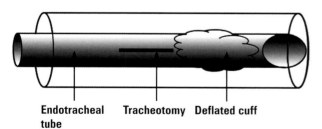

Endotracheal   Tracheotomy   Deflated cuff
tube

After Withdrawal of Endotracheal Tube

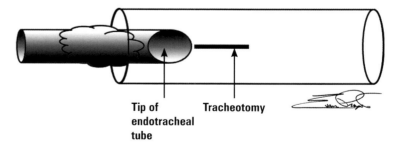

Tip of   Tracheotomy
endotracheal
tube

Step 17 Insert a 4.5-mm inner diameter cuffless PEDiatric tracheotomy tube (with obturator to make it slide more easily) into the tracheotomy stoma. Dunk it in saline first to make it slide into the trachea more easily.

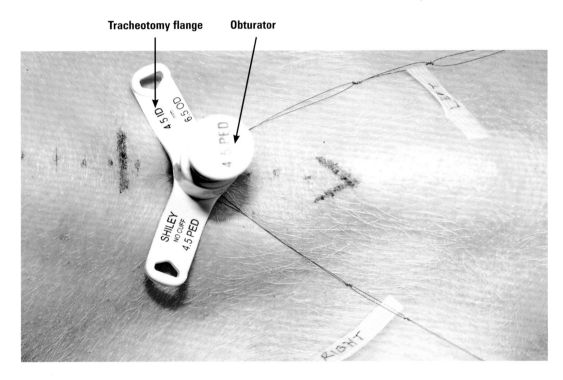

Tracheotomy flange   Obturator

Step 18 Remove the obturator quickly so the airway is not obstructed by it. Connect the anesthesia circuit to the tracheotomy tube. This does not have to be a sterile circuit—it is better to attach a nonsterile circuit than it is to search for a sterile circuit while the patient desaturates.

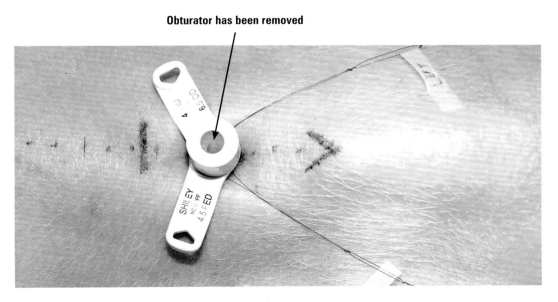

Obturator has been removed

Tracheotomy

There are many ways to secure a tracheotomy. Some surgeons suture the flanges to the skin. However, if the tracheotomy becomes plugged and cannot be unblocked, these sutures must be cut quickly to remove the blocked tracheotomy. Other surgeons cut the tracheotomy ties in half and cut small slits through the ends to allow the ties to pass through themselves. However, this weakens the ties and can cause them to rip. The method of placing tracheotomy ties described below avoids these issues. Ask your assistant to hold the tracheotomy in the airway while you place the ties.

Step 19 Pass the full-length tie through the hole in one tracheotomy flange. Pull it through until both ends are equal in length.

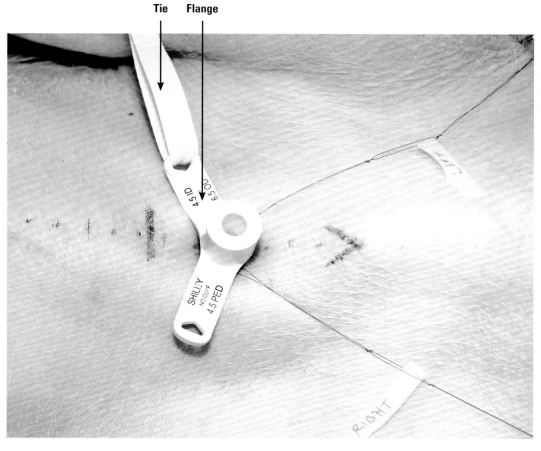

Tie   Flange

Anesthetic circuit has not been attached to allow full visualization of flanges and ties

Step 20 Pass both ties behind the neck. Make sure they do not twist or else they can cause a pressure sore. Place one tie through the hole on the other tracheotomy flange.

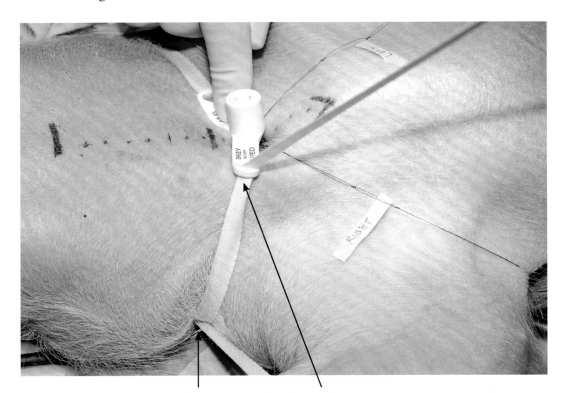

Both ties passed behind neck

One tie passed through other tracheotomy flange

Step 21 Ask your assistant to place his/her pinky finger under the tie (so it is not compressing the jugular vein) and tie one square knot that will not loosen. Only tie one knot at first, ask your assistant to remove his/her finger and gently pull on the tracheotomy. Ideally, the tracheotomy tube should be able to move anteriorly approximately 5 mm and not pull out of the tracheotomy stoma. The ties should not be so tight that they are constricting venous return. After you have reached these goals, tie the remaining knots in the ties so they do not slip.

KEY POINTS

Tie 1 square knot that will not loosen but not so tight that it will constrict venous return

Tie remaining knots and trim ties

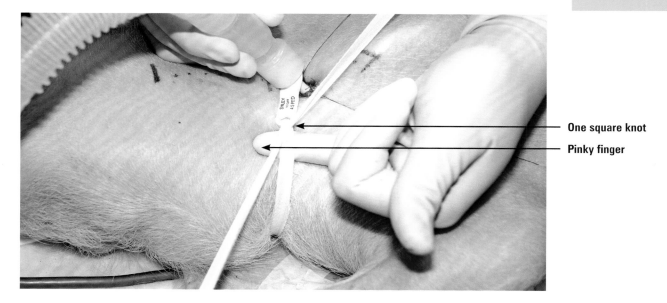

One square knot

Pinky finger

Step 22 Trim the ties.

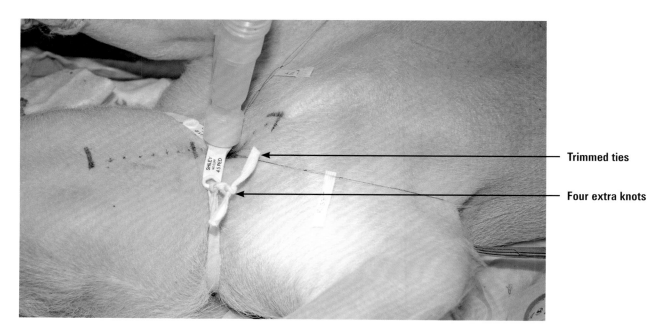

Trimmed ties

Four extra knots

12

Placing a Stent
(Double Stage)

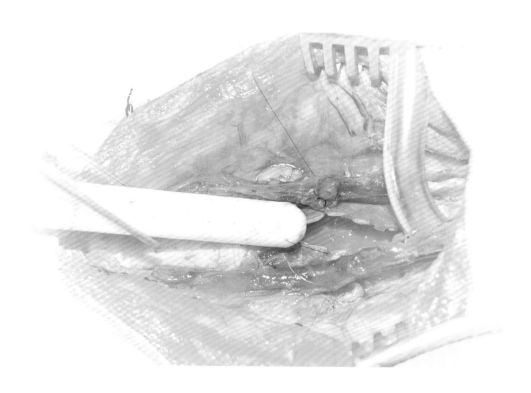

Disposable Items You Will Need

MEDICATIONS

- Akmezine
- Lidocaine 1% with 1/100,000 Epinephrine
- Pledget with oxymetazoline or topical epinephrine (4)
- Normal saline bag (3)

SHARPS

- 16- or 18-Gauge angiocatheter (2)
- 25-Gauge Butterfly needle (1)
- 25-Gauge angiocatheter (1)
- 27-Gauge angiocatheter (1)
- 2-0 Silk suture (9)
- 3-0 Polyglactin (Vicryl) suture (5)
- 4-0 Polypropylene (Prolene) suture on RB-1 tapered needle (5)
- 4-0 or 5-0 Polydioxanone (PDS) on RB-1 tapered needle
  OR Polypropylene (Prolene) suture on RB-1 tapered needle (9)
- 4-0 Poliglecaprone (Monocryl) suture (2)
- 3-0 Chromic gut suture on
  SH-1 tapered needle (4)
- #15 blade (1)
- #10 blade (1)
- Beaver blade (1)

OTHER

- 10 mL syringe (2)
- Intravenous tubing (1)
- 6.0 or 6.5 Cuffed endotracheal tube (1)
- Second endotracheal tube (cuffed 6.5 armored OR 7.0 oral RAE OR cuffed 6.5 regular tube)
- 11 mm airway stent (1)
- Gloves (2 pairs)
- Strip of material (30 cm)
- Absorbent pad (1)
- Rope (180 cm)
- Marking pen (1)
- Ruler (1)
- Green towel (8)
- Sterile adhesive strips (2)
- Penrose drain (2)

OPTIONAL

- 4.5 PED tracheotomy with ties (1)

Placing a Stent (Double Stage)

A stent is most commonly placed in the airway when a posterior laryngotracheoplasty using costal cartilage graft has been performed and the patient is scheduled to keep his or her tracheotomy postoperatively for a period of time until the repair has proven to have healed. This is called a "double-stage," "two-stage," or "staged" laryngotracheoplasty because the first stage is the airway reconstruction and the second stage involves removing the tracheotomy tube (i.e. decannulation). The stent prevents the posterior costal cartilage graft from migrating anteriorly into the airway. An anterior costal cartilage graft may also be placed in this situation.

In this porcine model, you will first need to perform a tracheotomy. *Human patients will likely already have a tracheotomy if you are planning to perform a double-stage laryngotracheoplasty.*

Step 1 Follow the steps outlined in "Tracheotomy." You may omit the step of inserting the tracheotomy tube if cost is an issue in this porcine model.

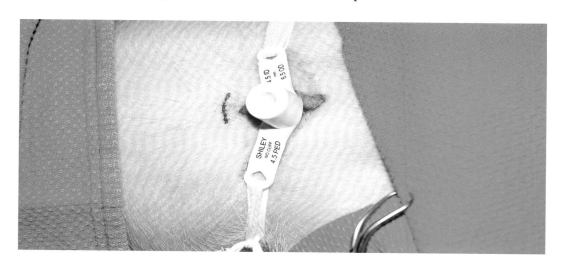

KEY POINTS

Endotracheal tube through tracheotomy stoma

RAE tube or cuffed armored endotracheal tube

Trim sharp edge

Create new Murphy eye

Place endotracheal tube

Suture to chest

Step 2   Replace the tracheotomy tube with an endotracheal tube placed through the tracheotomy stoma. There are two ways to do this. You may alter an oral RAE (Ring, Adair, Elwyn) tube, or you may use a cuffed armored endotracheal tube. To alter an oral RAE tube, cut a 7.0 endotracheal tube 4 cm away from the bend on the same bevel as the tip of the tube. Trim the sharp edge that is created. Create a new Murphy eye at the end of the tube.

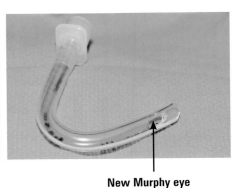

Scissors   Tip of endotracheal tube   Scissors trimming sharp edge

4 cm

New Murphy eye

Step 3   Place the newly created endotracheal tube into the tracheotomy stoma and suture it to the chest using 2-0 silk sutures.

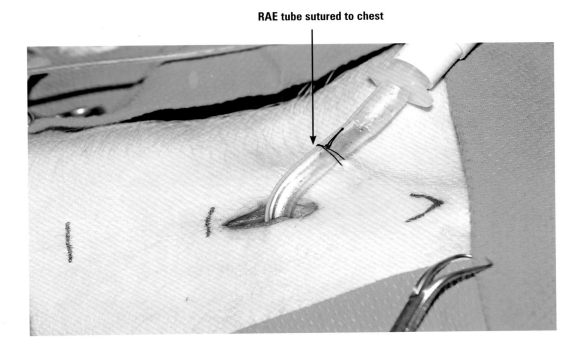

RAE tube sutured to chest

Step 4 Follow the steps outlined in "Exposure and Anatomy of the Pig Airway: Comparison with the Human Airway."

Step 5 Create a temporary tracheotomy lower down in the trachea by making a vertical incision through two tracheal rings.

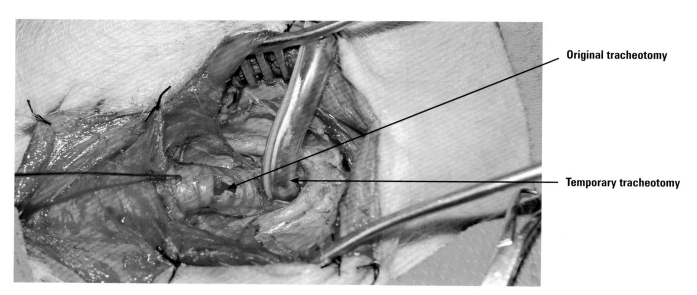

Temporary tracheotomy

Original tracheotomy

Step 6 Relocate the endotracheal tube from the original superior tracheotomy to the newly created temporary stoma and suture it to the chest with a 2-0 silk suture.

Original tracheotomy

Temporary tracheotomy

Step 7 Divide the cricoid cartilage and anterior tracheal rings vertically in the midline down to the original tracheotomy stoma. Measure the length from the superior aspect of this division to the superior aspect of the original tracheotomy stoma; this is the length of the costal cartilage graft that will be required.

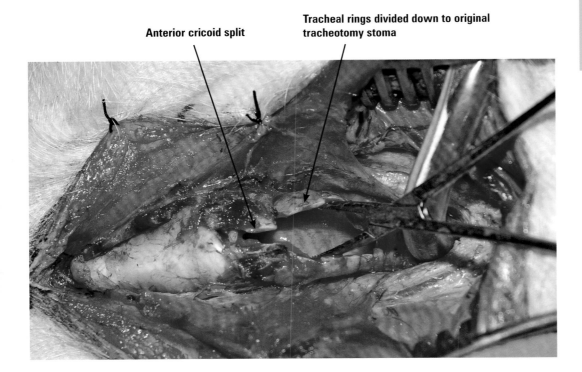

Anterior cricoid split

Tracheal rings divided down to original tracheotomy stoma

Step 8 Follow the steps outlined in "Harvest of Costal Cartilage Graft." If one rib is not long enough to provide two grafts of necessary length, harvest a second rib.

Step 9 Follow the steps outlined in "Posterior Laryngotracheoplasty Using Costal Cartilage Graft."

Step 10 There are many types of airway stents that can be used. Some of the more popular stents include the Aboulker stent (Pouret Medical, France), the Montgomery stent (Boston Medical, Massachussets), the Rutter Suprastomal stent (Boston Medical, Massachusetts), or a cut endotracheal tube. An Aboulker stent (11-mm outer diameter) works well in this porcine model because of cost issues. Orient the stent with the cap superiorly and place it into the airway to approximate the length required (superior edge of thyroid cartilage to superior edge of tracheotomy stoma). This length should be approximately 6.5 cm. It is better to overestimate the length and trim the stent later.

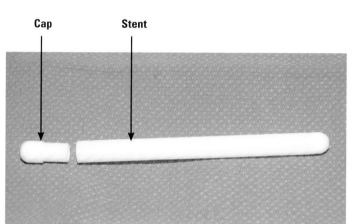

Cap   Stent

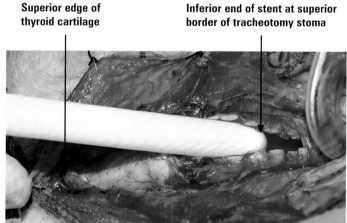

Superior edge of thyroid cartilage

Inferior end of stent at superior border of tracheotomy stoma

Step 11 Shorten the stent by removing the cap and cutting it 5.5 cm from the distal end. Place the cap on the new shorter stent.

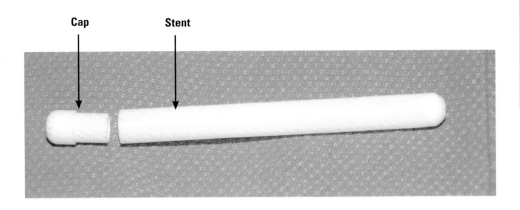

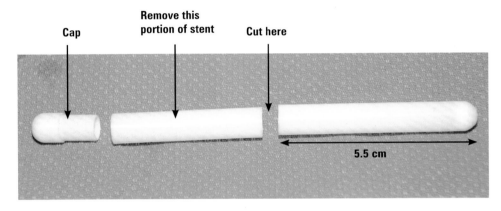

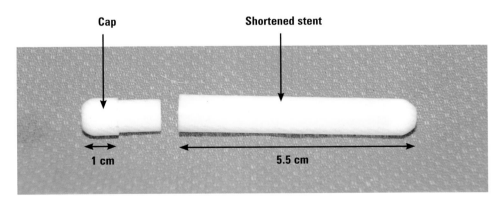

Placing a Stent (Double Stage)

12

Step 12   Place the stent into the airway and slide it superiorly through the vocal cords. Place a 4-0 Prolene suture through the left sternocleidomastoid muscle, the left sternohyoid and sternothyroid muscles, the left side of the trachea, and the inferior end of the stent just above the tracheotomy stoma.

KEY POINTS

Place stent in airway and slide superiorly through vocal cords

Secure with 4-0 Prolene suture

Place snap over both ends of suture to hold stent in place

Placing suture through stent

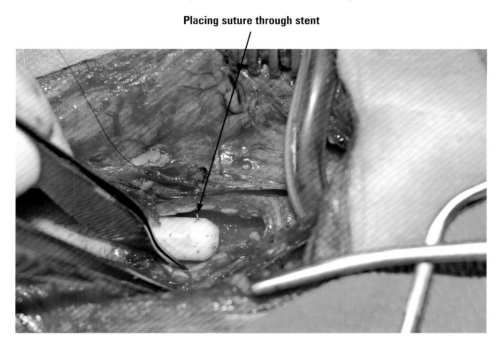

Step 13   Then pass the suture through the right side of the trachea, the right sterno-hyoid and sternothyroid muscles, and the right stenocleidomastoid muscle. Place a snap over both ends of the suture to hold the stent in place. The stent can now be moved in and out of the trachea while its inferior end remains anchored above the tracheotomy stoma.

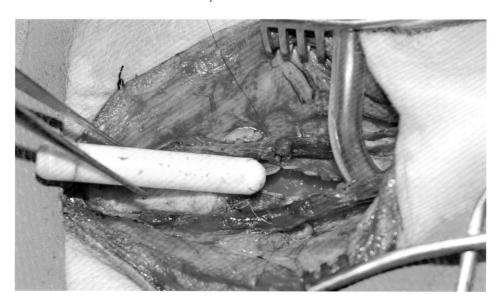

Step 14 *In humans, a rigid laryngoscopy is performed to visualize the position of the superior aspect of the stent. Ideally, stents with gentle rounded tips should reside midway up the epiglottis. If the stent is too long, it can be removed through the anterior aspect of the trachea, the cap can be removed, and the superior end of the stent can be trimmed. Keeping the inferior end of the stent anchored above the stoma with a suture allows you to trim the superior end of the stent and place it back where it was prior to trimming.* You may practice this maneuver in this porcine model if you wish.

Step 15 Measure the length of the defect from the superior edge of the cut cricoid cartilage to the inferior edge of the stent (superior edge of original tracheotomy stoma). This will be the required costal cartilage graft length. *In humans, if the cartilage around the tracheotomy stoma is soft and requires more support, convert the temporary tracheotomy stoma to a permanent one, and place the stent at the superior aspect of the new stoma with a cartilage graft covering the entire distance. Some surgeons advocate relocating all stomas to decrease the potential for infection and suprastomal collapse.*

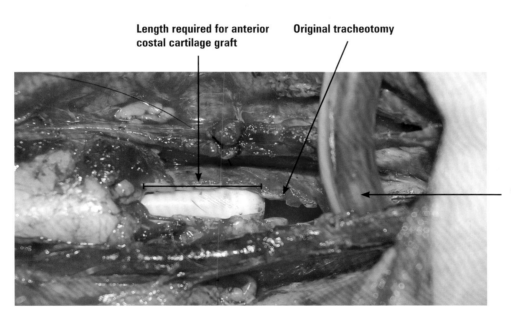

Length required for anterior costal cartilage graft

Original tracheotomy

Temporary tracheotomy

Step 16 *The rib in the pig is much thinner superiorly than it is in humans.* Cut off the thin superior edge of the graft to make it easier to carve flanges.

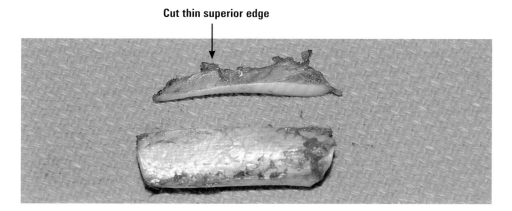

Cut thin superior edge

Step 17 Use a marking pen to draw an ellipse at one end of the graft on the anterior surface (perichondrial side). The other end of the drawing should be square. The length should match the measured length of the extended anterior cricoid split. The width should be as large as possible while allowing flanges to be carved, which in the pig is approximately 4 mm to 5 mm *(5 mm to 6 mm in humans)*. The flanges around the edges will be approximately 2 mm wide. Draw a line on the side of the graft denoting half the thickness of the graft.

Anterior Surface of Rib Graft

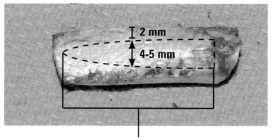

2 mm
4-5 mm

Length of extended anterior cricoid split

Side of Rib Graft

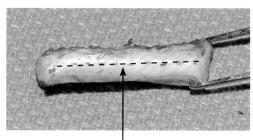

Line denoting half of the thickness

Step 18 Use a #10 scalpel to incise along the line denoting half the thickness of the graft to a depth of 2 mm. Repeat on the other side of the rib graft. Incise along the ellipse down to the level of the lateral cuts.

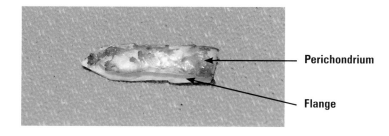

Perichondrium

Flange

Step 19 Suture the graft into the defect using either 4-0 or 5-0 sutures made of polydioxanone (PDS) or Prolene on a tapered needle. The benefit of the 4-0 suture is that it is less likely to break. Benefits of the PDS suture are that it has a bit of stretch to it that decreases the likelihood it will break when tying knots, and that it eventually resorbs after several months. The graft can be sutured with horizontal mattress sutures or simple interrupted sutures. We describe here the horizontal mattress suture technique.

A, Pass the needle through the tracheal cartilage from outside to inside, coming out submucosally on the lumenal side.
B, Pass the suture through the right angle formed by the flange and the graft.
C. Exit through the midline of the graft.
D. Pass the suture back through the graft and exit through the right angle formed by the flange and the graft.
E. Enter the tracheal cartilage submucosally passing from medial to lateral.

Snap the suture ends together. Try to make these suture ends equal in length by adjusting the suture length after each pass through cartilage rather than after passing through all of the cartilages. Pulling the suture through after passing through all cartilages risks tearing the cartilage.

KEY POINTS

Suture the graft using 4-0 or 5-0 sutures

Horizontal mattress or simple interrupted sutures

Sutures pass through lumenal side submucosally

Sutures pass through right angle formed by graft and flange

Pull suture through after each pass through cartilage

Horizontal Mattress Sutures

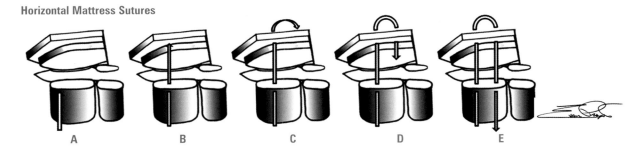

A   B   C   D   E

Proponents of horizontal mattress sutures believe that placing the suture knots laterally allows for the strap muscles to directly contact the new graft anteriorly for better revascularization. If you do not believe this theory, then you may use simple interrupted sutures to suture the graft in place.

Try to minimize the number of needle passes through the cartilage because each needle pass injures the chondrocytes in the graft. Each suture is pulled through until the two suture ends are even and a snap is placed to keep them together (tying the knots as you go makes it difficult to place additional sutures).

Step 20 Place sutures along both sides of the graft as well as superiorly. It is not as important to prevent an air leak in double-stage procedures as it is in single-stage procedures. In double-stage procedures, the air is more likely to leak around the tracheotomy tube than above it through a gap in the reconstructed airway.

Step 21 Arrange the "snapped" ends of the sutures neatly from superiorly to inferiorly. As one surgeon tightens each set of sutures from superiorly to inferiorly, the other surgeon allows the graft to "parachute" down into the defect. Tie the sutures with five to six knots. A Valsalva maneuver to check for an air leak is not required in a double-stage procedure.

KEY POINTS

Place sutures superiorly and along both sides of graft

Arrange "snapped" ends of sutures

"Parachute" graft into defect

Tie sutures with 5 to 6 knots

Anterior costal cartilage graft

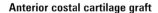

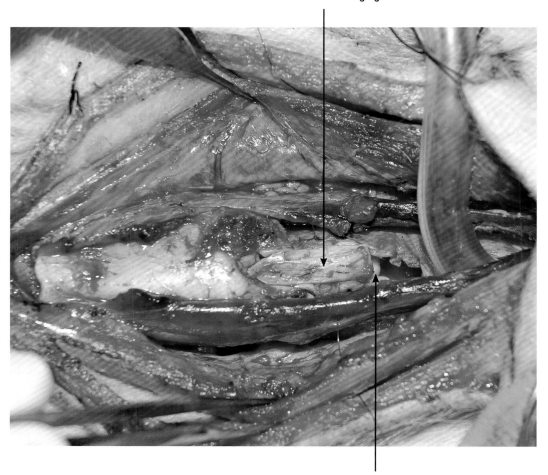

Stent

Step 22 Cut the end off of an 18-gauge angiocatheter (2 cm length) and place it over one end of the Prolene suture.

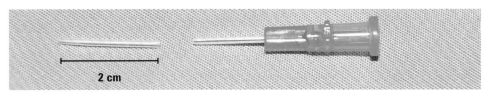

2 cm

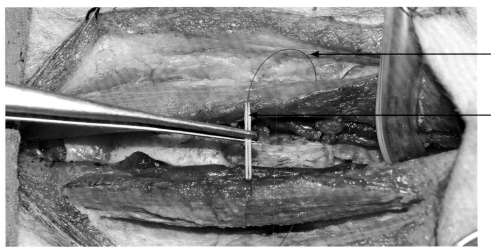

Prolene suture

Cut angiocatheter

Step 23 Tie the two ends of the suture together. Note how the angiocatheter prevents the suture from pulling through the sternocleidomastoid muscles. Tie numerous knots so that the long chain of knots extends toward the right side of the skin incision. This ensures that it will be easily found several months later when you reopen the neck incision, cut the suture and remove the stent during bronchoscopy under general anesthetic using endoscopic guidance. Alternatively, the sutures can exit through the skin on either side of the neck and be tied over a Silastic button. This makes removal of the sutures easier, but can introduce infection and the patient may manipulate the button.

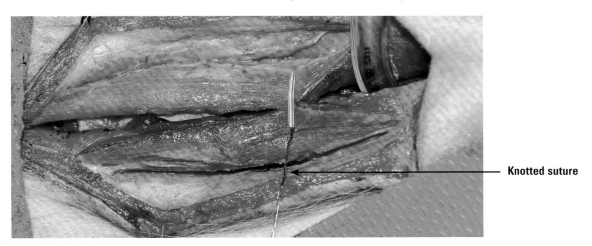

Knotted suture

Step 24 The distal temporary tracheotomy is sutured closed using 4-0 PDS or Prolene sutures.

Temporary tracheotomy sutured closed

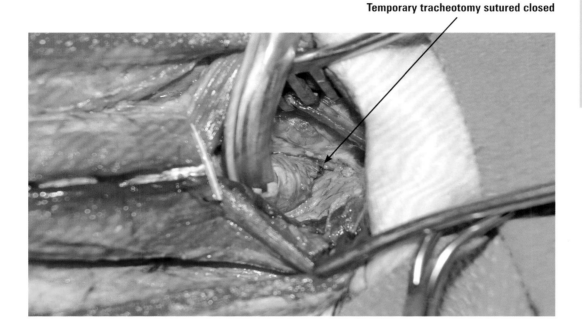

Step 25 *In humans, the wound is irrigated and tissue glue may be used over the closed temporary tracheotomy site and around the edges of the graft. However, we do not recommend wasting tissue glue while practicing on this porcine model. The skin is closed in layers and a Penrose drain is sutured in the corner using a 2-0 silk suture. The long chain of knotted suture securing the stent is placed as close to the right side of the incision as possible.* In this porcine model, suture the wound closed in layers and replace the endotracheal tube with the tracheotomy tube.

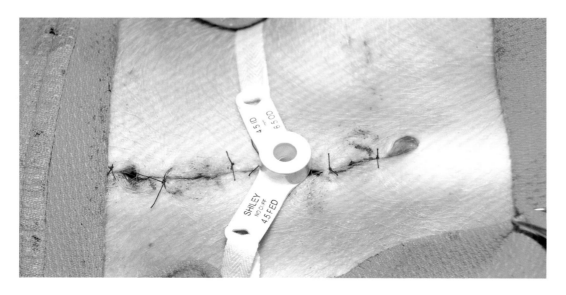

13

Cricotracheal Resection (Single Stage)

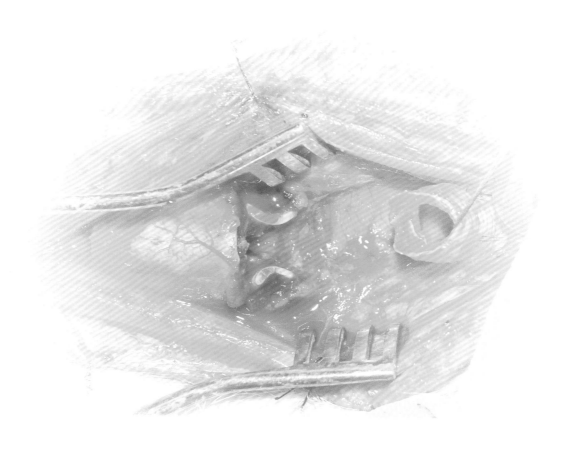

Disposable Items You Will Need

MEDICATIONS

- Akmezine
- Normal saline bag (3)

SHARPS

- 16- or 18-Gauge angiocatheter (1)
- 25-Gauge Butterfly needle (1)
- 2-0 Silk suture (7)
- 3-0 Polyglactin (Vicryl) suture on RB-1 tapered needle (2)
- 3-0 Polydioxanone (PDS)
  OR Polypropylene (Prolene) suture on RB-1 tapered needle (4)
- 4-0 Polydioxanone (PDS)
  OR Polypropylene (Prolene) suture on RB-1 tapered needle (1)
- For continuously running anastomotic suture:
  36-inch double-armed 4-0 Polydioxanone (PDS) on RB-1 tapered needle (1)
  OR 30-inch double-armed 5-0 PDS on RB-1 tapered needle (1)
- For simple interrupted anastomotic sutures:
  4-0 Polydioxanone (PDS)
  OR 4-0 Polypropylene (Prolene) on RB-1 tapered needle (10)
- 4-0 Poliglecaprone (Monocryl) suture on P-3 reverse cutting needle (1)
- #15 Blade (1)
- Beaver blade (1)

OTHER

- 10 mL syringe (1)
- Intravenous tubing (1)
- 6.0 or 6.5 Cuffed endotracheal tube (1)
- Second endotracheal tube (cuffed 6.5 armored OR 7.0 oral RAE OR cuffed 6.5 regular tube)
- Gloves (2 pairs)
- Strip of material (30 cm)
- Absorbent pad (1)
- Rope (180 cm)
- Marking pen (1)
- Ruler (1)
- Green towel (4)
- Penrose drain (1)

OPTIONAL

- Large McGowan needle (1)
- 24 or 26 Rusch Maloney esophageal bougie (1)
- 5 mm Diamond burr with drill (1)

Cricotracheal Resection (Single Stage) **13**

Step 1 Intubate with a cuffed endotracheal tube, but deflate the cuff when you enter the airway.

Step 2 Place a Rusch Maloney esophageal bougie (size 24 or 26, the smaller the better) into the esophagus to delineate it better when separating the trachealis muscle from the esophagus.

Step 3 Follow the steps outlined in "Exposure and Anatomy of the Pig Airway: Comparison with the Human Airway."

Step 4 Perform a temporary tracheotomy fairly low down in the trachea (between the eighth and ninth cartilaginous rings) so there is enough room to work comfortably in the upper airway. An armored endotracheal tube with the cuff deflated works well for this. You may also use a modified oral RAE tube, as demonstrated in "Placing a Stent" on page 94. However, a regular endotracheal tube will suffice if costs are a consideration. Place the endotracheal tube off to the left side of the chest. Suture it to the chest with 2-0 silk sutures.

KEY POINTS
Intubate

Place esophageal bougie

Temporary tracheotomy

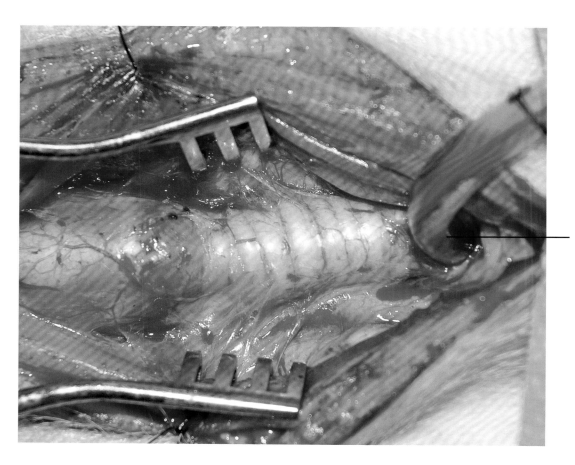

Temporary tracheotomy

Step 5 Place retention sutures into the distal trachea. This ensures that when the trachea is divided, the distal part does not fall away into the chest. Place two sutures (3-0 Prolene or PDS) into the anterior tracheal wall, one on each side. Keep the needle on the suture because you will need it later to wrap around the hyoid bone.

A. Pass the suture distally in the submucosal plane posterior to two tracheal rings.
B. Loop the suture anteriorly and proximally around the distal tracheal ring.
C. Pass the suture back proximally in the submucosal plane posterior to the proximal tracheal ring.

KEY POINTS

Place retention sutures

Protect yourself from needles

Retention Sutures

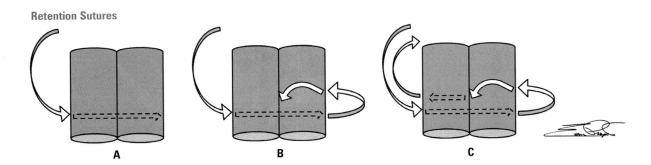

A   B   C

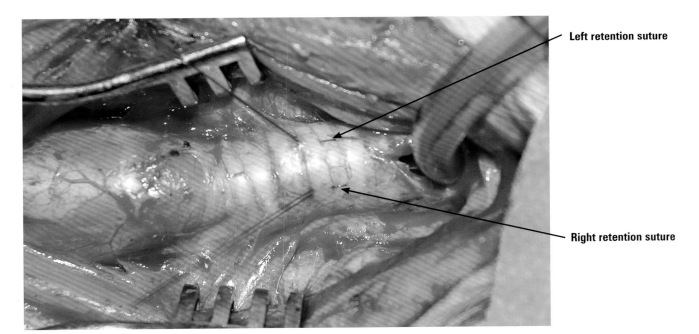

Left retention suture

Right retention suture

This technique will minimize the chance that the suture will pull through the cartilage. At the termination of the case, these sutures will be looped around the hyoid bone to act as internal Grillo (chin-to-chest) sutures. Protect these needles so you do not get injured during the surgery.

Step 6 Use a straight beaver blade to enter the airway with a small horizontal incision along the inferior border of the cricoid cartilage.

Cricoid hook   Cricoid cartilage   Horizontal incision

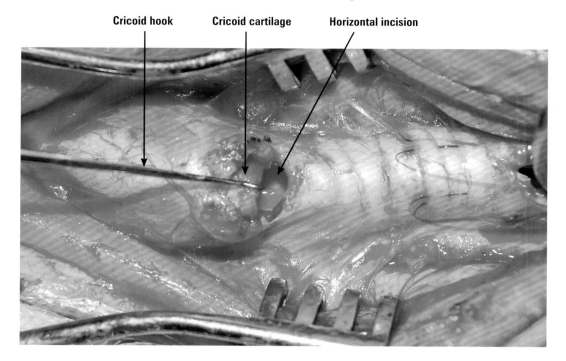

Step 7 *At this point in humans, you would inspect proximal to this cut to determine if the airway was stenotic. If it was stenotic you would divide the cricoid vertically in the midline.* In this porcine model, pretend there is stenosis and divide the cricoid vertically in the midline.

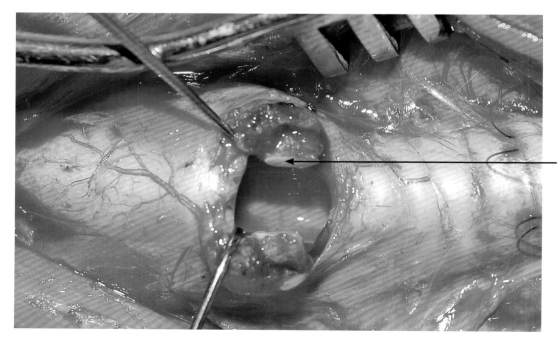

Divided cricoid cartilage

Step 8 *At this point in humans, you would inspect distal to this cut to determine if the airway was stenotic. If it was stenotic, you would divide the first tracheal ring vertically in the midline.* In this porcine model, pretend there is stenosis and divide the first tracheal ring vertically in the midline. *In humans, if the trachea is narrowed distal to this, divide more tracheal rings inferiorly until the airway is no longer stenotic.*

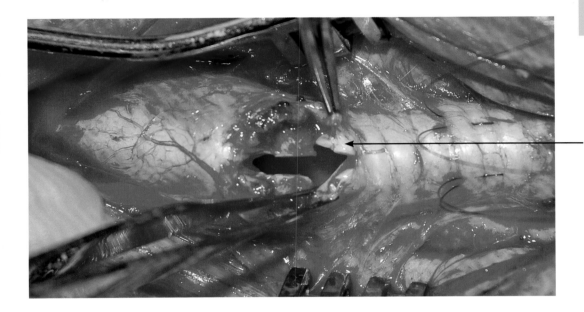

Divided tracheal rings

Step 9 There are many different ways to remove the cricoid and other narrow segments of the airway. The following method provides a safe way to remove the cricoid while minimizing the risk of injury to the recurrent laryngeal nerves. Using this method, remove the anterior aspect of the cricoid cartilage by making lateral cuts halfway between the anterior and posterior aspects of the cricoid. Care is taken not to make these cuts too far posteriorly so as to decrease the risk of injury to the recurrent laryngeal nerves. In a similar fashion, the anterior aspects of stenotic tracheal rings can be removed with lateral cuts.

KEY POINTS

Lateral cuts

Remove anterior aspect of cricoid and tracheal rings

Before

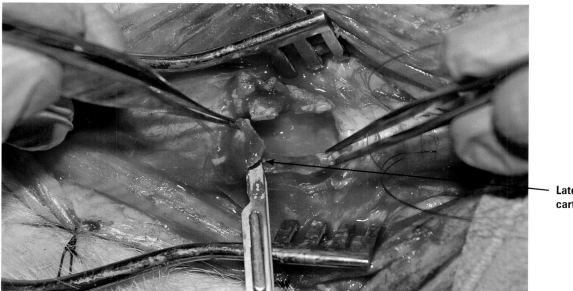

Lateral cut through cricoid cartilage

After

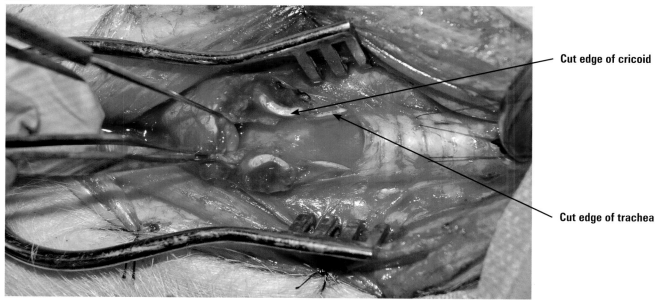

Cut edge of cricoid

Cut edge of trachea

Step 10 Use a scapel to incise the mucosa along the inferior border of the posterior cricoid plate. Use sharp scissors to divide the trachealis muscle.

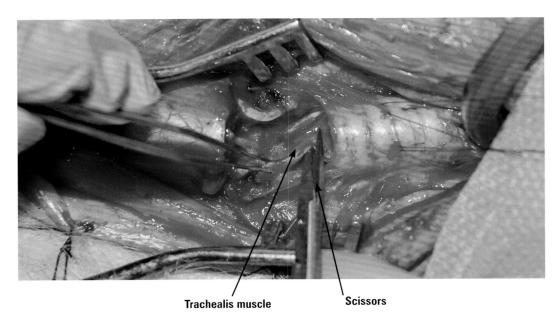

Trachealis muscle   Scissors

Step 11 Peel the trachealis muscle off the esophagus while trying to preserve the trachea's posterolateral attachments that are its blood supply. Gently sliding your finger between the trachealis muscle and the esophagus helps to dissect this plane nicely.

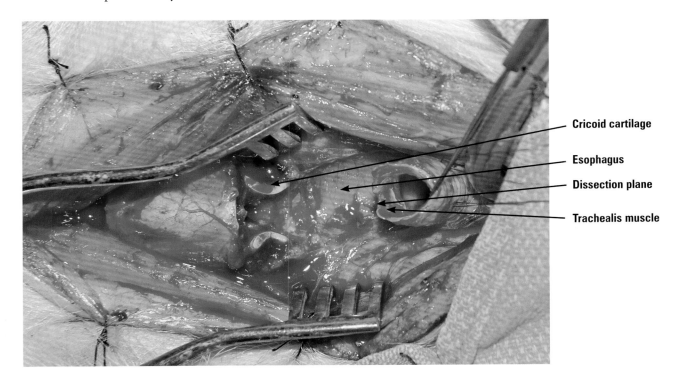

Cricoid cartilage

Esophagus

Dissection plane

Trachealis muscle

Step 12   Use a round knife (as is commonly used in middle ear surgery) or Freer elevator to elevate the mucosa off the posterior cricoid plate proximally. Remove the elevated mucosa by incising it sharply with a scalpel. This new mucosal edge will later become the superior edge of the anastomosis between the thyroid cartilage and the trachea.

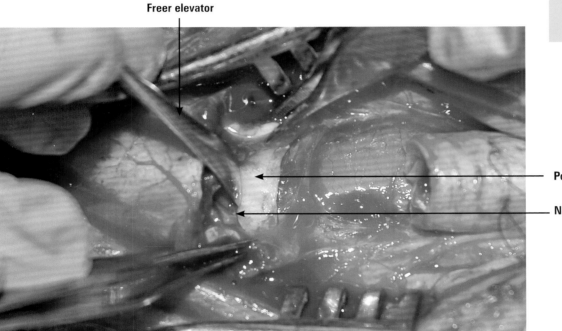

Freer elevator

Posterior cricoid plate

New mucosal edge

Cricotracheal Resection (Single Stage) 13

Step 13 *In humans, a 5-mm diamond burr is used to thin down the posterior cricoid plate. This allows the distal trachea to be pulled superiorly over top of it.* By thinning the cricoid plate well (also known as "eggshelling"), the lateral aspects of the posterior cricoid plate can be reflected posteriorly to protect the recurrent laryngeal nerves. Irrigate well while drilling so the recurrent laryngeal nerves do not get injured by the heat. This is best done by having one surgeon suction and drill while his/her assistant irrigates. If you do not have a drill in your animal facility, shave down the posterior cricoid plate using a #15 blade.

KEY POINTS

Thin the posterior cricoid plate

Reflect its lateral edges posteriorly to protect the recurrent laryngeal nerves

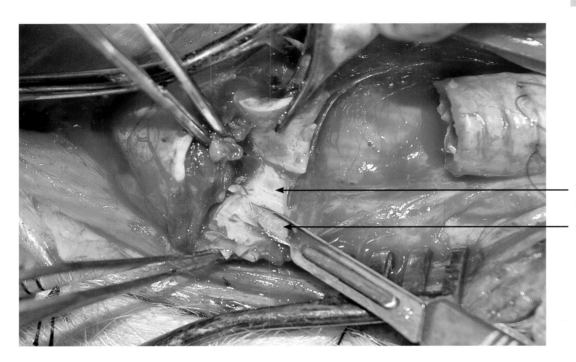

Thinning the posterior cricoid plate

Scalpel

Cricotracheal Resection (Single Stage)

13

Step 14 Place two additional posterolateral retention sutures (3-0 Prolene or PDS), one on each side of the trachea, to widen the posterior trachea as it slides superiorly into the posterior cricoid plate.

A. Pass the suture through the thyroid cartilage from outside of the lumen heading into the lumen but staying in a submucosal plane.
B. Traverse the gap and enter submucosally into the distal trachea, passing distally in the submucosal plane posterior to two cartilaginous rings (similar to the retention suture described in Step 5), loop anteriorly and proximally around the more distal ring, and pass submucosally along the posterior border of the more proximal tracheal ring.
C. Pass submucosally out through the thyroid cartilage.

Place a snap with a rubber shod (rubber tip to prevent tearing of the suture) on both ends of these sutures. A similar suture is placed on the other side of the thyroid cartilage and trachea.

KEY POINTS

Place two posterolateral retention sutures to widen the posterior trachea

A suprahyoid release helps close an anastomosis that would otherwise be under too much tension

Placement of Right Posterolateral Stay Suture

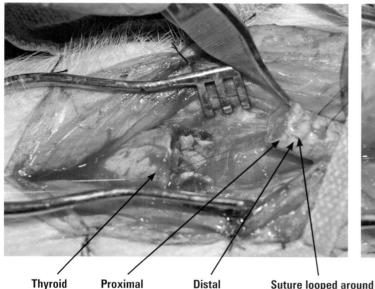

Thyroid cartilage | Proximal tracheal ring | Distal tracheal ring | Suture looped around more distal tracheal ring

Posterolateral Stay Sutures in Place

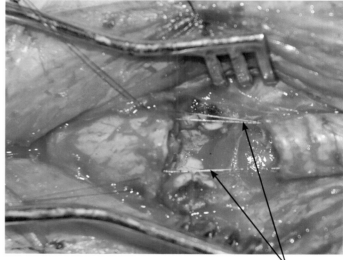

Retention sutures

Step 15 *In humans, if you need to resect a large amount of trachea that places the anastomosis under too much tension, a suprahyoid release can be performed.* In the animal facility, this porcine model does not require a suprahyoid release. However, you can practice performing a suprahyoid release by using the cautery to release the muscles from the superior aspect of the hyoid bone between the lesser cornua (horns). Use an elevator to find the subperiosteal plane to peel the remaining muscle off the bone.

Step 16   Pull the trachea superiorly over the thinned posterior cricoid plate. Gently tighten the stay sutures by pulling on them to hold these parts together.

Step 17   Join the thyroid cartilage and trachea using either a continuous running suture or multiple interrupted sutures. For the continuous running suture, a 36-inch double-armed 4-0 PDS suture on an RB-1 tapered needle (Ethicon) works nicely. Alternatively, a 30-inch double-armed 5-0 PDS suture on an RB-1 tapered needle (Ethicon) will suffice. Stand at the head of the bed facing the pig's feet.

A. Place the first stitch through the posterior wall of the trachea (from inside the lumen to outside).
B. Place the suture through the proximal aspect of the posterior cricoid plate and through the mucosal edge created in Step 12.
C. Pull the suture through halfway so both ends are of equal length.

KEY POINTS

Suture trachea to superior aspect of posterior cricoid plate

First stitch through posterior wall of trachea

Pull suture through halfway

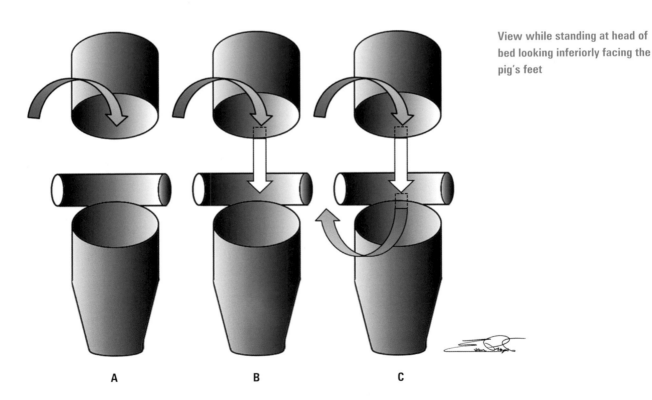

A   B   C

View while standing at head of bed looking inferiorly facing the pig's feet

Step 18 Run one end of the suture as an over-and-over baseball stitch up one side of the trachea and the other end of the suture up the other side of the trachea. Only suture the posterior half of the trachea. Place snaps with rubber shods (tips) over the needle to protect yourself, and do not cut them off—you will need them again later.

KEY POINTS

Suture over-and-over baseball stitch

Suture only posterior half of trachea

Place snaps with rubber shods over needle

Over-and-over baseball stitch along posterior half of trachea   **Trachea**   **Posterior cricoid plate**

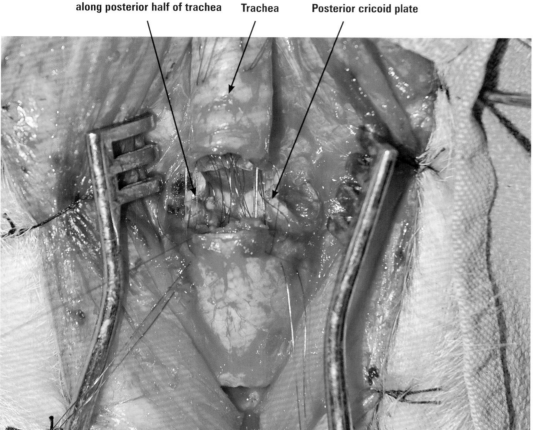

View while standing at head of bed looking inferiorly facing the pig's feet

Step 19 Tighten these sutures using two small blunt nerve hooks. Start posteriorly and work your way anterolaterally up each side in a hand-over-hand fashion. Do not release tension on the suture at any time.

Tightened suture along left side of anastomosis

Sutures along posterior wall of anastomosis

Tightened suture along right side of anastomosis

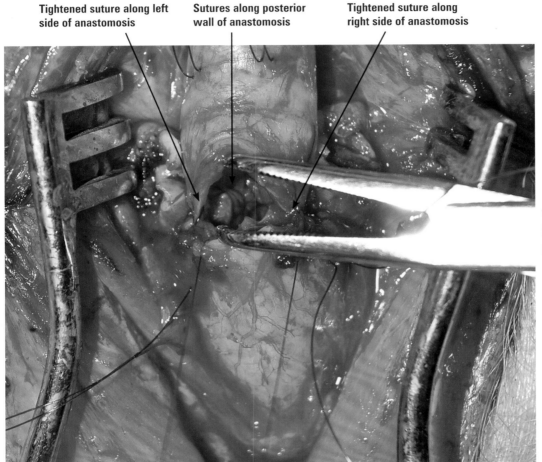

View while standing at head of bed looking inferiorly facing the pig's feet

Step 20 *A human patient would now be intubated nasally while the surgeon watches the endotracheal tube pass through the new anastomosis. The temporary tracheotomy tube is removed from the distal trachea. If a stent is to be placed in the airway for a double-stage procedure, whereby the patient will retain his or her tracheotomy, it is sutured in place at this time under direct visualization.* In this porcine model, reintubate orally, remove the temporary tracheotomy, and push the oral tube past the tracheotomy stoma.

Step 21 Continue the over-and-over baseball sutures around each side of the trachea until they meet in the midline. Tighten these sutures with two nerve hooks, as described in Step 19, and tie them together with six to eight knots. The sutures can be tied in one of two ways: (1) one suture exits the thyroid cartilage, the other exits the tracheal cartilage, and the two sutures are tied parallel to the pull of tension created at the anastomosis; (2) both sutures exit the same side (either thyroid cartilage or tracheal cartilage) and are tied perpendicular to the pull of tension created at the anastomosis.

KEY POINTS

Continue sutures anteriorly, tighten, and tie them together in the midline

Over-and-over baseball sutures tied in the midline parallel to the pull of tension created at the anastomosis

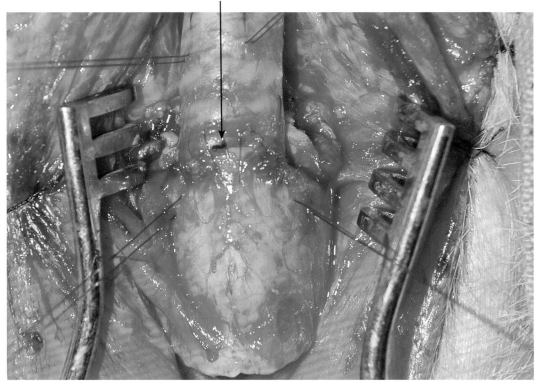

View while standing at head of bed looking inferiorly facing the pig's feet

Step 22 Tighten the posterolateral stay sutures to widen the distal trachea and pull it superiorly and posteriorly up into the thyroid cartilage.

KEY POINTS
Tighten posterolateral stay sutures

Loop anterior stay sutures around hyoid bone

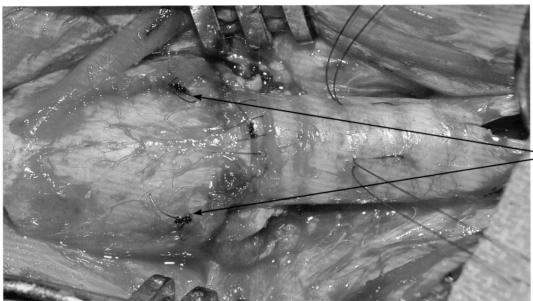

Posterolateral stay sutures

View while standing on the right side of the pig

Step 23 Loop the anterior stay sutures around the hyoid bone. These will take tension off the anastomosis in a manner similar to Hermes Grillo's external chin-to-chest sutures. *In humans, the hyoid bone can be quite large. The easiest way to place this suture is to pass a large McGowan needle (curved needle with an empty eyelet) partially around the hyoid bone, thread it with one end of the anterior stay suture, and then pull the threaded needle all the way through. In the piglet, the hyoid is smaller and the needle attached to the suture will pass around the hyoid bone.*

Hyoid bone   **Suture needle**

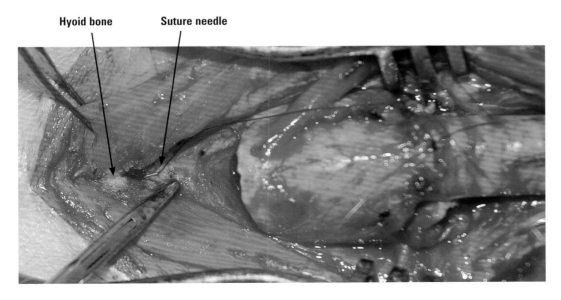

Step 24 Tie the suture. Repeat on the other side for symmetry.

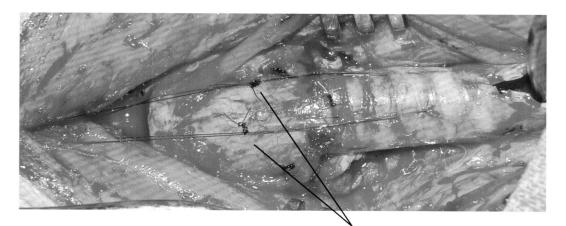

**Internal de-tensioning
Grillo sutures**

Step 25 Suture the temporary tracheotomy closed using interrupted 4-0 PDS sutures. *In humans, the wound is irrigated with antibiotic solution and a leak test is performed. Tissue glue may be applied over the anastomosis. A Penrose drain is placed in the right side of the neck wound. The wound is closed in layers with 3-0 Vicryl sutures, and the skin is closed with 4-0 Monocryl sutures. You may place either chin-to-chest sutures externally or a cervical collar to immobilize the neck to limit neck extension and decrease the risk of anastomotic dehiscence. A nasogastric tube is placed. A postoperative chest x-ray is performed to rule out pneumomediastinum.*

14

Slide Tracheoplasty (Single Stage)

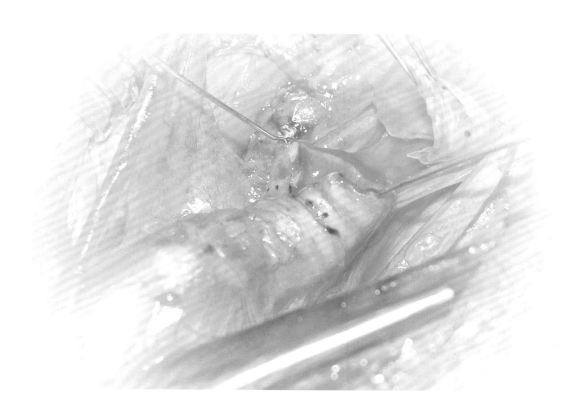

Disposable Items You Will Need

MEDICATIONS

- Akmezine
- Normal saline bag (3)

SHARPS

- 16- or 18-Gauge angiocatheter (1)
- 25-Gauge Butterfly needle (1)
- 25-Gauge angiocatheter (1)
- 2-0 Silk suture (7)
- 3-0 Polyglactin (Vicryl) suture on RB-1 tapered needle (2)
- 3-0 Polydioxanone (PDS) OR Polypropylene (Prolene) suture on RB-1 tapered needle (2)
- 4-0 Polydioxanone (PDS) OR Polypropylene (Prolene) suture on RB-1 tapered needle (1)
- For continuously running anastomotic suture:
  36-inch double-armed 4-0 Polydioxanone (PDS) on RB-1 tapered needle (1)
  OR 30-inch double-armed 5-0 PDS on RB-1 tapered needle (1)
- For simple interrupted anastomotic sutures:
  4-0 Polydioxanone (PDS) OR 4-0 Polypropylene (Prolene) on RB-1 tapered needle (10)
- 4-0 Poliglecaprone (Monocryl) on P-3 reverse cutting needle (1)
- #15 Blade (1)

OTHER

- 10 mL syringe (1)
- Intravenous tubing (1)
- 6.0 or 6.5 Cuffed endotracheal tube (1)
- Second endotracheal tube (cuffed 6.5 armored OR 7.0 oral RAE OR cuffed 6.5 regular tube)
- Gloves (2 pairs)
- Strip of material (30 cm)
- Absorbent pad (1)
- Rope (180 cm)
- Marking pen (1)
- Ruler (1)
- Green towels(4)
- Penrose drain (1)

OPTIONAL

- Large McGowan needle (1)
- 24 or 26 Rusch Maloney esophageal bougie (1)

Slide Tracheoplasty (Single Stage)

Slide tracheoplasty is a surgical technique used to widen a stenotic trachea. For simplicity, tracheal stenosis can be categorized as involving either the cervical or thoracic trachea. To perform a slide tracheoplasty on the thoracic trachea, the patient usually has to be placed on cardiopulmonary bypass and the procedure is performed without an endotracheal tube in the trachea. For the purposes of this pig dissection, we describe the steps involved in performing a cervical slide tracheoplasty with the piglet intubated through a temporary tracheotomy.

KEY POINTS

Intubate

Place esophageal bougie

Temporary tracheotomy

Step 1   Intubate with a cuffed endotracheal tube, but deflate the cuff when you enter the airway.

Step 2   Place a Rusch Maloney esophageal bougie (size 24 or 26, the smaller the better) into the esophagus to delineate it better when separating trachealis muscle from esophageal muscle.

Step 3   Follow the steps outlined in "Exposure and Anatomy of the Pig Airway: Comparison with the Human Airway."

Step 4   Perform a temporary tracheotomy fairly low down in the trachea (between the eighth and ninth cartilaginous rings) so there is enough room to work comfortably in the upper airway. An armored endotracheal tube with the cuff deflated works well for this. You may also use a modified oral RAE tube as demonstrated in "Placing a Stent" on page 94. However, a regular endotracheal tube will suffice if costs are a consideration. Place the endotracheal tube off to the left side of the chest and suture it to the chest with 2-0 silk sutures.

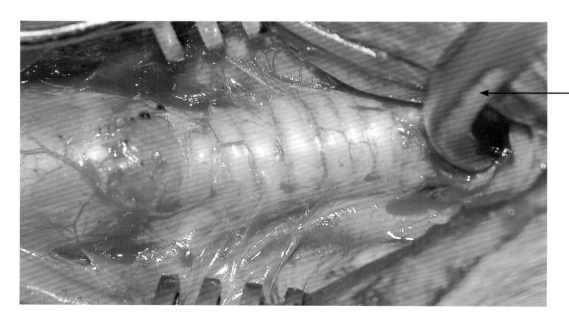

Temporary tracheotomy

Step 5 Place retention sutures into the distal trachea. This ensures that when the trachea is divided, the distal part does not fall away into the chest. Place two sutures (3-0 Prolene or PDS) into the anterior tracheal wall, one on each side. Keep the needle on the suture because you will need it later to wrap around the hyoid bone.

A. Pass the suture distally in the submucosal plane posterior to two tracheal rings.
B. Loop the suture anteriorly and proximally around the distal tracheal ring.
C. Pass the suture back proximally in the submucosal plane posterior to the proximal tracheal ring.

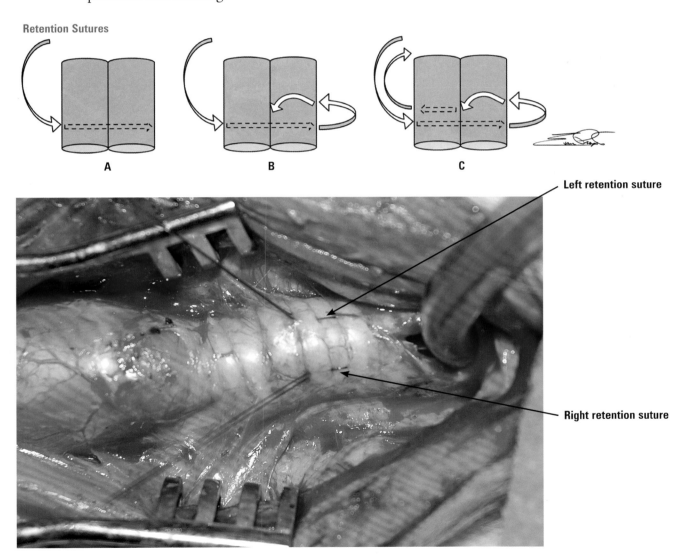

This technique will minimize the chance that the suture will pull through the cartilage. At the termination of the case, these sutures will be looped around the hyoid bone to act as internal Grillo (chin-to-chest) sutures. Protect these needles so you do not get injured during the surgery.

Step 6 *In humans with a thoracic tracheal stenosis who are intubated, a flexible bronchoscope is passed through the endotracheal tube and flexed anteriorly to touch the tracheal mucosa at the site of the stenosis. Turning off the overhead lights in the operating room will allow you to see the light from the scope so you can mark the site of stenosis with a marking pen. Alternatively, a 25-gauge needle can be placed through the trachea and visualized with the flexible scope to delineate the stenosis more accurately. In humans with a cervical tracheal stenosis who have a temporary tracheotomy, a rigid bronchoscope may be used instead of a flexible bronchoscope.*

KEY POINTS

Delineate site of stenosis with flexible or rigid bronchoscope

Use light or needle

Mark borders and middle of simulated stenosis

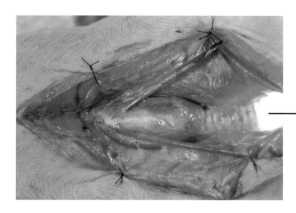

———— **Light from flexible bronchoscope**

Step 7 Many animal facilities do not have a bronchoscope. Therefore, for this pig dissection, mark two dotted lines on the trachea to simulate the length of a stenotic segment and place a single dot halfway between these lines.

Proximal end of stenosis

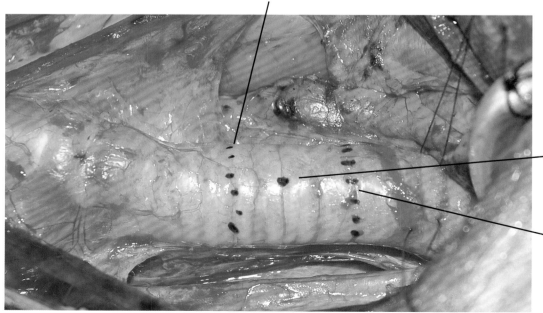

Single dot marking halfway point between dotted lines

Distal end of stenosis

Step 8 Dissect the trachea circumferentially between the dotted lines taking care not to injure the recurrent laryngeal nerves near the tracheoesophageal groove. The recurrent laryngeal nerves tend to course more laterally the further inferiorly you dissect in the chest. Use blunt dissection to separate the trachealis muscle from the esophagus and be careful not to enter into the trachea from posteriorly through the trachealis muscle.

Step 9 Use sharp scissors to divide the trachea on a bevel. The bevel can angle from antero-superior to postero-inferior or from antero-inferior to postero-superior. We show here the antero-superior to postero-inferior bevel because it is easier to suture the trachea back together using this method while standing at the head of the pig's bed. Start cutting between cartilaginous tracheal rings and cut across rings as you cut posteroinferiorly. It is easier to perform the next steps while standing at the head of the pig's bed facing the pig's feet.

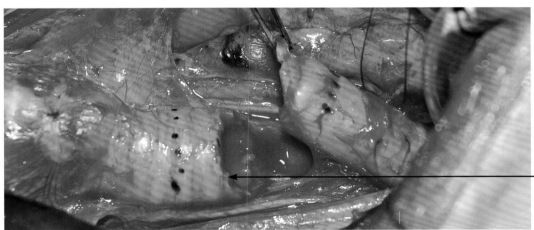

View while standing on the right side of the pig

Trachea divided on bevel

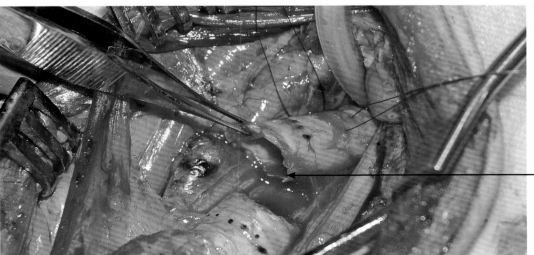

View while standing on the right side of the pig at the head of the bed facing the pig's feet

Trachea divided on bevel

Step 10 Divide the proximal tracheal rings *(which would likely be complete tracheal rings in a human)* anteriorly up to the proximal dotted line. Divide the distal trachealis muscle *(which would likely be complete tracheal rings in a human)* posteriorly down to the level of the distal dotted line that is marked on the anterior aspect of the trachea. These divisions will create new triangularly shaped edges.

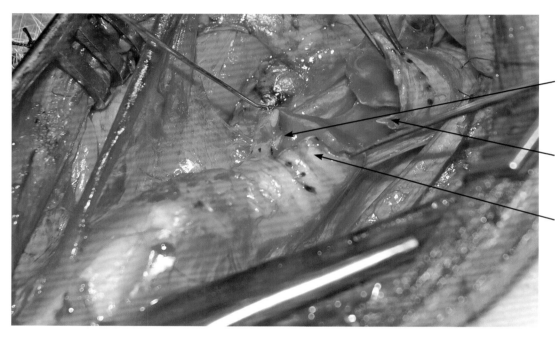

Divided proximal tracheal rings anteriorly

Divided distal trachealis muscle posteriorly

Newly created triangularly shaped edge

Step 11 Trim off the triangularly shaped edges on both sides of the proximal anterior tracheal division.

Scissors

Proximal anterior tracheal division

Triangularly shaped edge

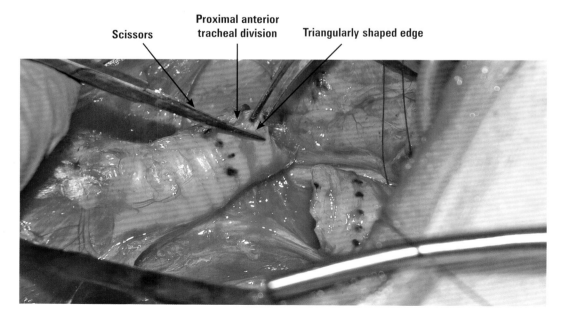

Slide Tracheoplasty (Single Stage)

14

Step 12 Trim off the triangularly shaped edges on both sides of the distal posterior tracheal division.

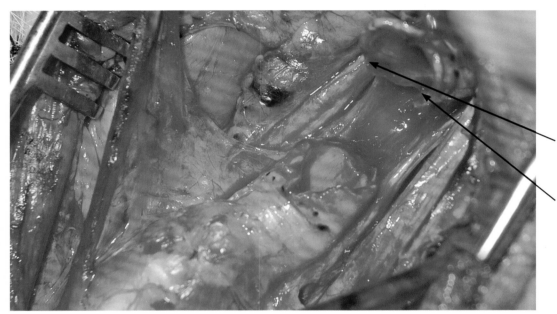

KEY POINTS

Trim off triangularly shaped edges of distal posterior tracheal division

Dissect trachea off of esophagus

Leave posterolateral blood supply

Triangularly shaped edge

Distal posterior tracheal division

Step 13 Dissect the proximal and distal parts of the trachea off the esophagus using sharp scissors and blunt finger dissection. Try to leave most of the posterolateral muscular attachments intact to preserve the tracheal blood supply.

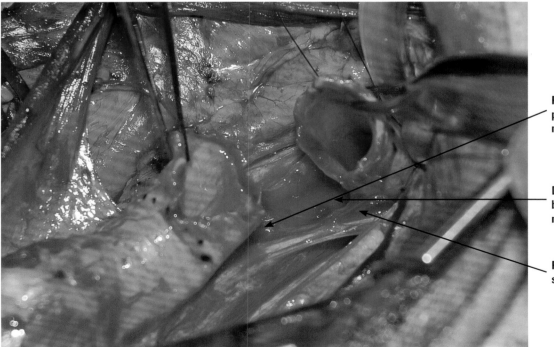

Proximal dissection plane between trachealis muscle and esophagus

Distal dissection plane between trachealis muscle and esophagus

Posterolateral attachments supplying blood to trachea

KEY POINTS

Suture distal and proximal trachealis muscles

Pull suture through halfway

Step 14 The trachea can be reapproximated using either a continuous running suture or multiple interrupted sutures (be sure to place the knots outside of the tracheal lumen). Because the technique of placing interrupted sutures is self-explanatory, we describe here the continuous running suture using a 36-inch double-armed 4-0 PDS suture on an RB-1 tapered needle (Ethicon). Alternatively, a 30-inch double-armed 5-0 PDS suture on an RB-1 tapered needle (Ethicon) will suffice. Stand at the head of the bed facing the pig's feet.

A. Place the suture through the apex of the distal posterior trachealis muscle (starting inside the tracheal lumen and heading outward posteriorly toward the esophagus).
B. Enter the proximal posterior trachealis muscle (heading from the esophageal side into the tracheal lumen).
C. Pull the suture through halfway so both ends are of equal length.

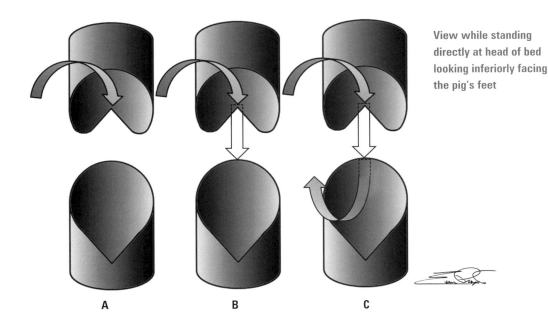

View while standing directly at head of bed looking inferiorly facing the pig's feet

A   **B**   **C**

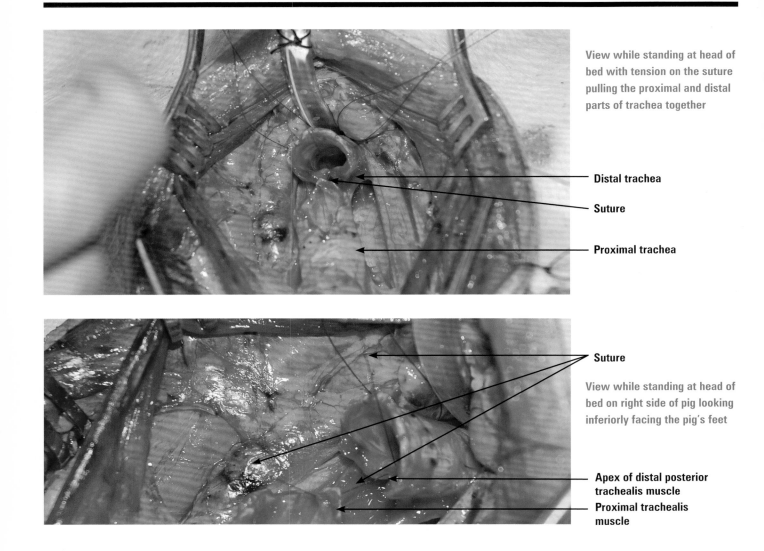

View while standing at head of bed with tension on the suture pulling the proximal and distal parts of trachea together

Distal trachea

Suture

Proximal trachea

Suture

View while standing at head of bed on right side of pig looking inferiorly facing the pig's feet

Apex of distal posterior trachealis muscle

Proximal trachealis muscle

Step 15 Use the suture from the distal tracheal lumen to run an over-and-over baseball stitch up the left side of the trachea. Place a snap with a rubber shod (tip) on this suture needle to protect yourself.

KEY POINTS

Run suture up left side of trachea

Run suture up right side of trachea

Only suture posterior half of trachea

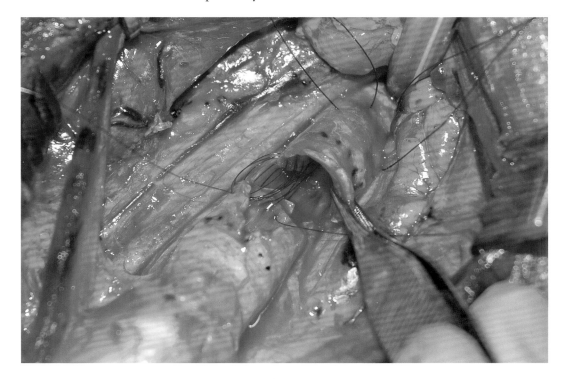

Step 16 Use the suture from the proximal tracheal lumen to run an over-and-over baseball stitch up the right side of the trachea. Place a snap with a rubber shod (tip) over this suture needle to protect yourself. Only suture the posterior half of the trachea.

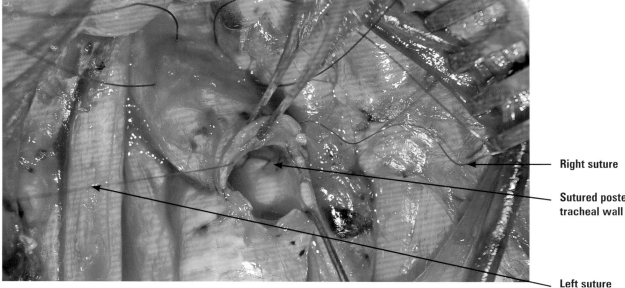

Right suture

Sutured posterior tracheal wall

Left suture

Slide Tracheoplasty (Single Stage)

14

Step 17 Use two small blunt nerve hooks to tighten the sutures in a hand-over-hand fashion. Start posteriorly in the midline and work your way anterolaterally around each side. To do this, place one hook under one suture loop, pull gently, then maintain tension on this loop while the other hook tightens the suture loop next to it. Continue doing this first up the left side and then up the right side of each tracheal wall.

Step 18 *In a human patient, you would now reintubate the patient nasotracheally to minimize endotracheal tube movement postoperatively.* In this porcine model, reintubate orotracheally.

Step 19 Continue the over-and-over baseball sutures around both sides of the trachea anteriorly. Tighten these sutures with nerve hooks and tie them together with six to eight knots.

KEY POINTS

Use blunt nerve hooks to tighten sutures

Reintubate nasotracheally in humans and orotracheally in pigs

Run sutures around anterior trachea and tie them together

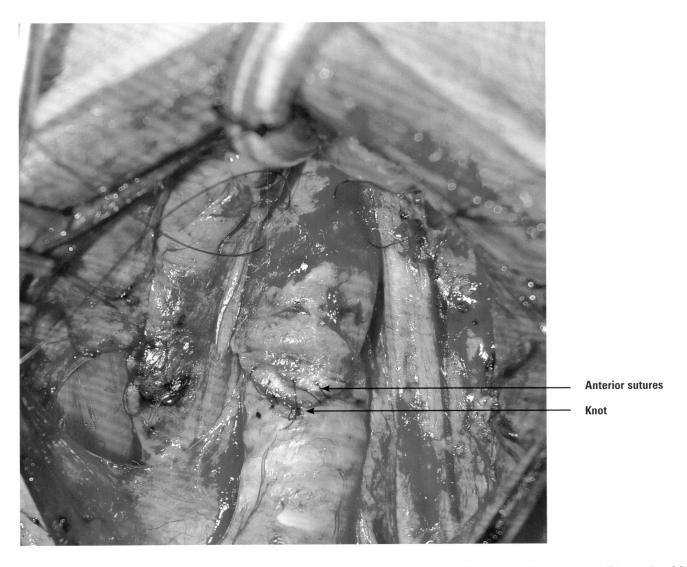

Anterior sutures

Knot

Slide Tracheoplasty (Single Stage)

14

Step 20 Because you are performing a cervical slide tracheoplasty, place internal sutures to take tension off the anastomosis as is performed in a cricotracheal resection. De-tensioning sutures are not commonly used in a thoracic slide tracheoplasty.

Loop the anterior stay sutures around the hyoid bone. These will take tension off the anastomosis in a manner similar to Hermes Grillo's external chin-to-chest sutures. *In humans, the hyoid can be quite large. The easiest way to place this suture is to pass a large McGowan needle (curved needle with an empty eyelet) partially around the hyoid bone, thread it with one end of the anterior stay suture, and then pull the threaded needle all the way through.* In the piglet, the hyoid is smaller and the needle attached to the suture will pass around the hyoid bone.

KEY POINTS
Loop anterior stay sutures around hyoid bone

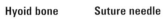
Hyoid bone   Suture needle

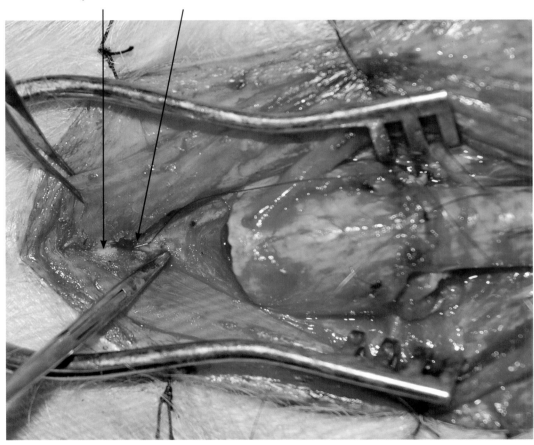

De-tensioning sutures used in cervical slide tracheoplasty are similar to those used in cricotracheal resection shown here

Airway Reconstruction Surgical Dissection Manual   **137**

Step 21 Tie the suture. Repeat on the other side for symmetry.

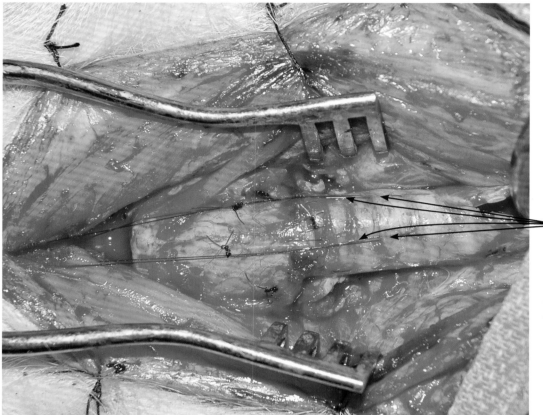

Internal de-tensioning Grillo sutures

De-tensioning sutures used in cervical slide tracheoplasty are similar to those used in cricotracheal resection shown here

Step 22 Suture the temporary tracheotomy closed using interrupted 4-0 PDS sutures. *In humans, the wound is irrigated with antibiotic solution and a leak test is performed. Tissue glue may be applied over the anastomosis. A Penrose drain is placed in the right side of the neck wound. The wound is closed in layers with 3-0 Vicryl sutures and the skin is closed with 4-0 Monocryl sutures. You may place either chin-to-chest sutures externally or a cervical collar to immobilize the neck to limit neck extension and decrease the risk of anastomotic dehiscence. A nasogastric tube is placed. A postoperative chest x-ray is performed to rule out pneumomediastinum.*

Index

Index

Stay suture, 83
Stenotic airway, 111
Stenotic trachea, 127
Sternal, 17
Sternal notch, 15, 77
Sternocleidomastoid muscle, 16
Sternohyoid muscles, 78
Sternothyroid muscle, 17
Sternum, 41
Straight iris scissors, 4
Subperichondrial flap, 30
Subplatysmal flap, 16
Suprahyoid release, 117
Surgical instruments, 4

Suture, 36, 58, 102, 110, 118

T

Thyroid ala cartilage graft, 35
Thyroid cartilage, 15, 17, 19, 23, 29, 35, 55
Thyroid gland, 19
Tongue, 8
Towel clip, 4
Trachea, 19, 81
Trachealis muscle, 114
Tracheal lumen, 25
Tracheal rings, 23, 35, 55, 112

Tracheal stenosis, 127
Tracheotomy flange, 86
Tracheotomy, temporary, 63, 93, 95, 109, 127
Tracheotomy ties, 87

V

Valsalva maneuver, 37, 51, 59, 69
Ventriculoperitoneal shunt, 41

X

Xiphoid process, 42